Three Generations
Fight Cancer Together

Lessons Learned on the Journey

ELAINE GREYDANUS BUSH

Published by EA Books Publishing a division of
Living Parables of Central Florida, Inc. a 501c3
EABooksPublishing.com

"Through an honest and humble account of her journey through the darkness of cancer, Elaine beautifully articulates the importance of choosing. Choosing each day to stay focused on Jesus, allowing Him to renew and infuse us with His joy, hope and peace, oftentimes in unexpected ways."

Kristen Ward
Daughter of a Breast Cancer Victim

"Powerful! Wonderful writing, clear, precise, and intriguing sweeping the reader into the intense story of a family's journey. This book provides a guide that will help and inspire others facing their own battles. The stories evoke emotions and reflections for the reader. Elaine's grandchildren add their thoughts and actions which provide unique encouragement and insights. *Three Generations* delivers hope to those struggling with life's concerns and difficulties."

Susan M. Brems
M.Ed, Retired Teacher

"Another title for this beautiful, heartfelt book might be *You are not Alone*. Because that is clear from Elaine's words and counsel. As the wife of a cancer patient, she draws on deep reservoirs of faith and grace as she journeys along with Wayne, their children, and grandchildren through the landmines of cancer. Readers whose family members have been affected by cancer will be encouraged, blessed, and nurtured by this warm, wise and Scripture-rich book. Most of all, they will find in Elaine a dear companion who reminds them that they are never by themselves, even on the hardest emotional expeditions of their lives."

Lorilee Craker
Author of "Anne of Green Gables, My Daughter and Me: What My Favorite Book Taught Me About Grace, Belonging and the Orphan in Us All"; "Money Secrets of the Amish," "Through the Storm" with Lynne Spears and "My Journey to Heaven" with Marv Besteman.

"Elaine touches the heart of a family faced with the anguishing reality of cancer. Through her warm, conversational style, she shares her passionate faith, nurtured since childhood through critical life experiences. Cancer creates ripples. Its radius affects much and many, as I know from my brother's fight with cancer. Praise God for the amazing ways He works in our lives!"

Fayth Steensma
Sister of a Cancer Sufferer

"Captivating! A compelling narrative of faith and hope. Three generations together weave a tapestry of love and support for one another as they journey with cancer, an unwelcome companion. This book does indeed "bear witness" to the faithfulness of our God and the peace and hope that is ours in Christ Jesus."

Kathy Richert
Cancer Survivor

DEDICATION

To:

Our children, who would not let us travel alone;

Our grandchildren, who loved us with their prayers,
hugs, cards, drawings, and words;

My husband Wayne, who walked through
this fire with courage and grace;

And to our God, who fights for us, we bear witness:
He is faithful!

Dear Reader,

You are not alone. I share our story to assure you of that and in the hope of encouraging you who are unwillingly drafted into this war. Shared stories can help make the battles of life bearable. Knowing I am not the only one who sometimes feels so stunned and inadequate for the task at hand, and hearing how someone else made it, provides ideas and strategies I can use.

The American Cancer Society estimates that in 2016 there were over 1,685,000 people diagnosed with cancer in the United States. For many of them, like our family, the diagnosis is a bombshell with a lot of collateral damage. The word *cancer* explodes in the heart of the patient. Its sound waves shatter the peace of the family spreading out to stun loved ones and friends, reaching neighbors, acquaintances, and beyond. Our fight began the year my husband was diagnosed with a rare cancer. Our battle brought us on a marathon through unknown territory.

There was good news: God was with us. He shed light for one step at a time and revealed his love in unexpected and detailed ways. Our children and grandchildren volunteered to join forces with us against the enemy that assaulted Wayne's body and all of our emotional and spiritual fortresses.

People often ask, "What can I do?" This book offers some answers through the lessons we learned of what was helpful, and how we could help each other. The story is woven with the past, because that is how we became the family who grew stronger during the long conflict.

Our story is not exactly like anyone else's, but there are similarities. We are ordinary people who have experienced the disappointments, challenges, and joys of life. My prayer is for you, traveling this unexpected journey. Know that God is at work within us and for us, even on the battlefield of cancer.

Trust Him,
Elaine

We will tell the next generation the praiseworthy deeds of the LORD, His power, and the wonders He has done. Psalm 78:4

For You I Write

I am writing to you
the one on the singular journey
the one who has stepped off the path

you know who you are
you desperately want to know
has anyone been this way before

you search for flares, flashes of light
scan the horizon for signals, sparks
evidence that you aren't the first to walk this way

a burning bush takes your breath
woos you off the broad path
and plunks you on a narrow way

others saw the same bush
were curious like you
inquired, began

For you I write
leaving a trail of words
so you know
you are not alone.

Sharon Ruff
Used by permission

CONTENTS

Three Generations

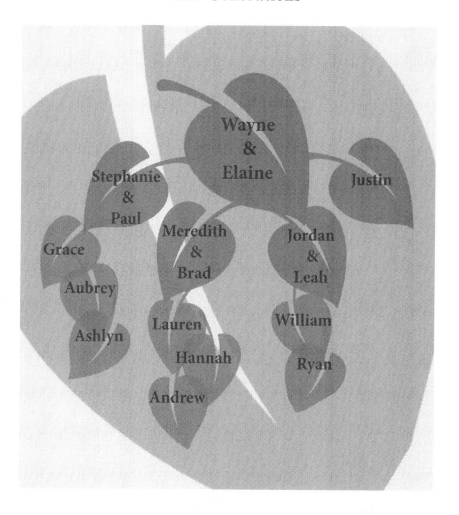

Chapter 1

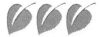

Our World Tips

In this world you will have trouble . . . . John 16:33

The sleet ticked against the window. It was the end of January, the evening of a winter-gray day in Michigan. Supper dishes were done; we had eaten something though neither of us had felt like it lately. When the phone rang I jumped, tense from waiting.

"Can you get Wayne on an extension? I want to talk to both of you." The doctor's voice was flat, heavy.

"It's Doc. He has news." Wayne didn't look at me. He seemed frozen, sensing the report that would change our lives.

*****

The problem had started a month earlier during Christmas week; minor, not worth mentioning. Later, he would tell me it was just an ache, like a pulled muscle. But on New Year's Eve it persisted and finally three nights later it woke him up and kept him up. As soon as the doctor's office opened, I called, and they told us to come right in.

In all our years of marriage, I had rarely gone with Wayne to a doctor's appointment, but something nudged me to go with him this time.

"Doctor would like *you* to come in," the nurse called me as I sat in the waiting room. Wayne's physician had just examined him. I found myself clenching my teeth, a habit I have tried to replace with a deep breath. I put the unread magazines back on the end table.

"I'm concerned this might be a hernia that needs surgery," he began. I had heard of that. My shoulders dropped, some of the tension released. But then he paused and added, "I'm not sure, so I'm scheduling an ultrasound. That will give us more information." His eyes had been on Wayne, but then he turned to me, his voice no longer objective, "I love Wayne like a brother; I'll take good care of him."

Wayne looked at me; I reached for his hand.

I remember the first time I held Wayne's hand. It was much younger then, unsullied by the passage of time and hard work. It was only two months after a friend had pointed him out to me as he left the high school cafeteria. "He's cute, don't you think? He's a twin. They look a lot alike." That's my earliest memory of seeing Wayne. It wouldn't be long before I was timing my walk from one class to the next so our paths would cross. Sometimes it meant lingering at my locker, risking the dreaded tardy bell. I disappointed my regular babysitting clients for a Friday night basketball game, willingly choosing to give up added savings for college just to watch him play, and for the few minutes we could chat when he left the locker room headed for his ride home. We were sophomores at Eastern Christian High School in New Jersey.

I wasn't sure he was as smitten with me as I was with him. He was friendly with everyone, but then in late fall of that year we went on a scavenger hunt. I managed to get on his team. It was a blustery cold evening. My ski jacket had no pockets so I resorted to tucking my freezing hands under my arms. Seeing my awkward efforts Wayne generously offered one of the oversized pockets of his cargo jacket. Delighted, I accepted. He soon slipped his hand into the same pocket and wove his fingers through mine.

By the end of our junior year I wrote in my diary, *I don't know if I'll marry Wayne Bush, but whoever does will be lucky, he's one of the nicest people I know.* I was the lucky one; years later, I married him.

*****

Two days after the initial doctor visit, Wayne was scheduled for an ultrasound which resulted in a quickly-scheduled CAT scan.

"Looks like serious inflammation, but I'm not sure of the cause. We need more tests. I've also called the urologist. You have an appointment in two days. Will you be able to make it?" Was there a choice, a doubt? Fear was beginning to gnaw at our sleep and peace.

The new doctor was professional and efficient. While he examined Wayne, I waited in the hall and tried to muster up a positive attitude. *OK, find out what's wrong and fix it. Lots of people get hernias and doctors know how to deal with them.* My mind searched for what else could be wrong in that area, but my limited medical knowledge came up empty. Self-talk quickly proved ineffective; faith regained ground so I prayed: *Please, God, give this doctor some wisdom and the answers Wayne needs, and please keep me calm and encouraging. Stop my racing thoughts.* I would lift these requests many times in the months ahead.

Finally, the doctor opened the door and waved me in. He sat down, paged through a pile of medical sheets, and began, "It's not your prostate or . . ." (a list of organs I no longer remember). With each "It's not" my hope increased. Then the sledge hammer, ". . . but your right kidney is beginning to shut down. I'll have to insert a stent from the kidney to the bladder and . . ."

"How long will it have to be there?" Wayne interrupted.

"Well, probably while you have chemotherapy." He paused as he saw our faces. "You understand it's probably cancer, right?"

No, no we didn't understand! That word, that awful punch-to-the-belly, take-your-breath-away word had not been uttered. How on earth had we gone from a possible hernia to a dysfunctional kidney to cancer?

He kept talking, ". . . schedule as soon as possible . . . I'll talk to your doctor, schedule a biopsy...."

We walked to the car. The sun was shining, but the world had changed. Before we pulled out of the parking lot, we sat, stunned. Finally, I touched Wayne's arm and whispered, "God help us. Please."

Pondering

Have you ever gotten unexpected news that stunned you? How did you react? Where did you find comfort? What helps? Have you ever wanted to pray, but couldn't find words?

Chapter 2

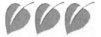

Waiting

I waited patiently for the Lord; He turned to me and heard my cry. Psalm 40:1

January 16, the middle of the month. Biopsy scheduled in three days, meanwhile Wayne was feeling better, no pain. We had told our children, "Dad is having some problems and is having tests." We tried to shield them from our deepest fears. Wayne was relieved to go off to work for the day: demolition and remodeling, physical work. Something he had begun in retirement. The doctor had said, "Do what you can." Good advice because we were in that difficult place, on hold, just waiting. The physical work done with one of his best friends, Nels, gave his day some laughter and distractions.

While he was out renovating old rooms, I went to a prison where a Shakespeare Behind Bars class was also doing some restoration, in this case, of broken lives. Six months earlier I had retired from teaching English at Calvin Christian High School. I missed the students, not the paper work, so I began to pursue other interests. A friend had invited me to go to the prison class. In spite of the hour drive each way and the stringent process needed to enter the prison, I found myself drawn to it. Shakespeare Behind Bars is a unique program that offers inmates the opportunity to study Shakespeare, perform his plays, and wrestle with the personal and social issues introduced in the stories.

Dressed in drab blue prison garb, the inmates came into the room pausing to smile and acknowledge each other. My tension melted on the first visit as one by one they greeted me with a warm handshake and,

"Hi, my name is___. Glad you're here." Eventually there were twenty or more prisoners sitting in a circle with a leader and a few of us visitors. My role was just to be there and be supportive.

The men memorized parts, and their ability to deliver difficult lines with articulation and passion at first startled me, and then became a source of enjoyment. Often, they discussed the motives of the characters. One day the leader asked, "Why did Brutus kill Caesar if Caesar was his friend?"

These men, some incarcerated for years already, were not only wrestling with the characters' motives. During a pause, one prisoner turned to me and asked why I thought he had joined his friends in an armed robbery when he knew it was wrong. "I've had a lot of time in here to wonder about that."

Startled by all eyes turned to me, I lifted a silent "Help me!" prayer and then reverted to the role of teacher. God brought to mind a high school lesson I had taught. "You, like Brutus, had a choice to make. Think about it: Why do we do what we do . . . any of us?"

"Consider this idea: Our beliefs and values lead to our behavior. It seems likely that your belief in being law-abiding clashed with the behavior your friends demanded. Because you valued your friends and their approval more than you valued the law, you changed your belief and convinced yourself that crime was okay, at least in that situation."

"Brutus did that as well. He said his love for his country clashed with his love for his friend Caesar because of the choices Caesar made in governing. A choice had to be made. What did he value the most: his friendship or his country?"

"What you believe and value will determine how you live."

It was quiet for a moment, then he nodded, smiled, "Yeah, what do I value?"

On my ride home I thought, *What do I value?* My boat was rocking by threats of cancer. I had choices to make. I had chosen to pray, and now I had another choice to make: Call in the troops.

*****

When you become a mom, a new type of love explodes. I still remember holding our first born, Stephanie, in the delivery room. I had longed for her arrival, eager to become a mom, taking all the classes, reading the books. What I was not prepared for was the intensity of protective love that burst in me the moment I held her. I knew I had suddenly turned into a mama bear who would do anything to protect this precious gift. That burst of almost over-whelming, protective love repeated when Meredith, then Jordan, and finally Justin arrived.

Even when Stephanie as an infant kept me walking her for hours—walking, not rocking, not sitting, just walking—at night while Wayne worked late, or when Justin as a one year old wanted to play for three hours in the middle of the night after ear infections woke him up, and I thought, *If you can die of sleep deprivation, I may not make it.* I loved them beyond anything I could fathom.

It did not diminish much, this protective love, as they became adults. I learned to hold it in check, but it is part of who I am. It gave me a little better understanding of how much God loves each of His children. That instinct made me want to soften the reports we were getting. I was to learn a lot from our kids, when I finally shared the unedited news.

Pondering

What do you value, believe? How do your values impact the choices you make and the way you live? Have you ever made a choice that violated your values? What happened?

What do you do when you are waiting for possibly difficult news? Do you edit information to your family and friends?

Chapter 3

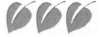

Sharing the News: Through their Eyes

Carry each other's burdens, and in this way you will fulfill the law of Christ. Galatians 6:2

I used to try to teach the idea of perception in school. It is a hard concept for teenagers to wrap their brains around. Truth is, it is hard for adults to understand. How often I have wondered, or more accurately, judged other people with condemning thoughts of: *What are they doing? What were they thinking? How can they act like that?* Even having taught perception, I can forget that each of us has our own unique load of experiences. Therefore, our own unique prism of memories through which we filter information and which influence our reactions to life.

To help my students *get it*, I would ask for three volunteers. Three fun-loving performers would come to the front of the class. I whispered instructions to them and one would disappear into the hall. The other two would begin to pantomime two friends talking. Suddenly the third volunteer burst into the room on all fours, barking. One of the friends ran away, and the other went to *pet the dog*. Why the different reactions? One had been bitten by a dog and perceived danger, and one only knew of friendly pets. Every individual reacts uniquely based on his or her own prism of memories.

I wasn't sure how our family would deal with this growing threat of cancer. All I could do was pray for them and trust that God would walk with each one of them. What began as Our Journey—Wayne's and mine—quickly became theirs as well, in spite of my protective love.

9

Once again I had to ask Jesus to give me His way of looking at people. Each one in the family had a unique perception of the situation.

Justin, our youngest, recalls, *I remember first thinking something might be more serious when Mom told me that Dad had seen the doctor and was getting more tests to see what was wrong. I remember thinking we usually share prayer requests, but this was different. Mom's tone of voice was different.*

As the days passed and he learned that it could be cancer: *I didn't know how to react. As selfish as this might come out, I was in such an emotionally low place from trying to accept my divorce, I didn't know how I could handle both blows at that time. I think I denied the thought of how serious cancer is. I have one of the closest families that is so blessed — this isn't possible. News like this doesn't happen to our family. If it is cancer, it'll be treatable.*

It is painful for me to read his words. We as a family had grieved deeply when Justin's marriage of five years had ended. As his mom, I had prayed and watched and often wept as he tried for over a year to save what was so precious to him, and to us. Justin's faith and grace had ministered to my heart, but I knew the scars he carried and the pain I could not lift. But God, even in this, His grace was evident. I witnessed that in Justin's life. How I longed to spare him more anguish.

Justin is our youngest, an unexpected addition whose life brought me to my knees and taught me a life-changing lesson. The lesson really started when I was pregnant with Jordan, who is two and half years older than Justin. In my seventh month of pregnancy with Jordan, a seizure in the middle of the night left me unconscious for over three hours.

Wayne called 911 at 2 a.m. and I was taken to the hospital. At 6:30 a.m. I remember hearing my doctor's voice asking if I could hear him or see him. "I can hear you, but I can't see you." For thirty minutes he stayed close by, trying to reassure me. I still remember praying over and over: *God, three little ones of yours need me. Please restore my sight.*

Finally, shifting light became shapes and gradually visual clarity returned. For three days I lay in a hospital bed waiting for answers, praying. Wayne was holding my hand when the neurologist came in to give us the results of a myriad of tests. Explanation: Not sure. The baby seems fine and there is no sign of a brain tumor—their first guess. They would monitor us and schedule a C-section which seemed the best way to deliver.

I adjusted to taking medication, being less confident of being in control, and relinquishing my driving privileges for a time. When Jordan was delivered healthy and sound, we were over the moon with joy, and I happily settled into the busy life of a mother of three. There were lingering effects. One was a loss of self-confidence, and another one continued to nag me even after almost two years. I was tired and couldn't seem to ever feel rested.

We had always wanted a big family, but it just did not sound like such a good idea anymore. I had been warned that another seizure during pregnancy or delivery could cause serious problems and possibly even death. So, reluctantly, we had decided to stop with three children. But God had other plans for us and a powerful lesson to teach me.

After months of increasing fatigue and spotty periods, I called my doctor to talk about a tubal ligation. Before the appointment, he wanted me to have a pregnancy test, just routine. Friday afternoon at 4 p.m. his nurse called. "Elaine, you're pregnant. . . . Did you hear me? Doctor would like you to come in on Monday. . . . Are you there? . . . Are you okay?"

Wayne found me hunched over on the floor in the living room, stifling my sobs, the phone still clenched in my fist. I could hear Stephanie, Meredith, and twenty-two month old Jordan playing in the family room.

"What? What is it?" He sat on the floor and rocked me.

"I'm pregnant! How could I have let this happen? I'm on anti-seizure medication, birth control pills, no prenatal vitamins."

"It's okay. It's going to be okay." He whispered and held me. "Go upstairs. I'll keep the kids busy."

How would I take care of this baby and the other three — if I lived? Would the baby be already impacted by my stupidity? I had been a speaker for Right-to-Life, and I felt like the devil was shaking me by the throat, mocking me: *So, what do you say now, you pro-lifer?! Your baby may be handicapped, and you won't even be around!*

The weekend felt like a boxing match I was losing. I was pummeled by fears, regrets, dread of the future. I tried to hide it from the kids, but Stephanie, who had just turned seven, would ask me, "What's wrong Mom?" I gave weak excuses. Wayne took over and gave me time to wrestle with the demons poking and prodding my faith, my peace, my hope. I wept into my pillow and cried out to God. I was exhausted but couldn't sleep, wallowing in my worries. Wayne felt my anxiety but did not share it. He reassured me that we would get through this together.

Monday afternoon I sat in Dr. B.'s office watching smiling moms in various stages of pregnancy go in for their appointments. Finally, I waited alone, his last patient, probably his most troubled that day. He had been there to help me through the long seizure and safely delivered Jordan. I was counting on him to help me through this.

His calm voice broke through some of my distress. He explained the risks both to the baby and me. He said the heartbeat was strong and I was already sixteen weeks along. He understood my disbelief, guilt, and fears. He also knew I would give my life for this baby. I would not consider abortion. When I left the office an hour later, I thanked God for a Christian doctor who would do all he could for us.

But as I drove home I continued to challenge God: *Why did you do this to this little one? —to our family? Where is the joy that there should be for new life?* He stopped me in mid-complaint: *Elaine, I made this baby. Can you love and care for him . . . for me?*

I looked at the passenger seat. No one there I could see, but I had heard the voice, the words, the question. *Can I love and care for this baby for you? Of course I will.* I said those words aloud, and at that moment, in a twinkling, peace and joy replaced every ugly fear. The burst of mother love that had exploded when Stephanie, Meredith, and Jordan were placed in my arms at birth, happened at that instant and filled every corner of my heart with love for my unborn baby.

It may be difficult to believe, but I can only tell you what I experienced, and it changed me. It was one of the hardest, but dearest lessons, I ever learned. My perception of who God is, how personal He is, how much He loves me, and how involved He is in the details of my life, took on new dimensions from that moment. I was reminded that I am ultimately not in control. Better by far to trust the One who is.

When I got home Wayne noticed the change in me. We gathered the children and told them the happy news. God had made a new life, and He was going to give that life to our family.

I thanked God each morning for creating this child and entrusting him or her to me. I would always include part of Psalm 139 in my prayer: *You are creating this little one in my womb, knitting this baby together. I praise you because he is fearfully and wonderfully made; your works are wonderful, I know that full well. His frame is not hidden from you as you make him in the secret place. You are weaving his unformed body together. All the days of his life are ordained by you and were written in your book before one of them came to be. How precious to me are your thoughts, O God!*

God was creating this new life, and He had created a new attitude in me. It seemed to be evident on my face. I discovered that in August when I was in my seventh month. We took a twelve hour car trip to Camp of the Woods in New York State to meet up with some of my family. As we were packing to come home, a husband and wife from a cabin near us stopped by. "We've been watching your family this week. We can't remember ever seeing a woman with three little ones and expecting another looking so . . . I don't know . . . joy-filled." I had to laugh. Only God could do that, change a terror-stricken woman into a joy-filled one.

Justin was born by C-section six weeks later, healthy, delightful; beloved by his father, siblings, and forever-changed mother.

*****

Jordan, a busy lawyer, husband, father, was also sorting through the information I was sharing. He recalls: *I remember thinking it was not going to be a big deal. There seemed to be so many other more likely, less serious explanations: a stomach bug, a hernia, an infection or even a benign mass. I did not want to worry too much until we knew there was actually something to worry about. This changed during a phone call with my sister when she commented, "J, I have a bad feeling about this." That was the first time the possibility of something more serious hit home.*

Leah, Jordan's wife, had already experienced serious health threats in her family. She had walked alongside them and shared her perspective: *I remember, to be honest, that I was not very concerned early on. Having gone through the experience of my sister's heart attack, I felt that if doctors were checking on him and they were doing so many tests that they would figure it out. I didn't want Mom or Dad B. to go through so much anxiety, so I was just praying the diagnosis and answer/plan would hurry up and get here.*

Brad, Meredith's husband, recalls: *Meredith and I had a sense that something was wrong without receiving the news. We knew that you probably had some information that we didn't and were trying to protect us as any parent/grandparent would do. We've known throughout this that you had a right to process information before relaying it on to anyone else, including us. We tried to respect that, but also show our care and concern throughout the process. I think even when we know something is wrong, we have a foundation that sustains us. God has been good to us throughout our lives and given us two sets of parents who modeled faith through all things. That being said, we hadn't been through anything like this before, so part of our faith is due to the fact that we've never had to go to this level of worry and dependence on God. We've never truly had to cry out for strength.*

After I had texted that it could be cancer: *Even in the thought of cancer, we rested in the fact that "God will care for us" and "medicine is incredible." Again, we were nervous and scared, but we didn't really go to that dark, dark place.*

13

The shield I had so carefully constructed to protect the family from worrying was disintegrating. We needed them. We needed their prayers, their love, and their presence. I was to learn many lessons on this journey; some I thought I knew, but it's funny how much better you learn a lesson when it becomes personal. I had to humble myself to ask for prayers, for support.

I wrote in my journal: *This week we have been living under the shadow of cancer. Wayne has had many tests in the last ten days. Words like* concerned *and* probably cancer *and* chemotherapy *have rattled our spirits and taken us from bed at 3 in the morning. "But yet . . ." Words from scripture. God is faithful. We have cried out to Him and (finally) asked family and a few close friends to pray for wisdom, peace, and healing. God is good. He has restored some peace, calmed our fears down, reminded us that this is no surprise to Him. Keep our eyes on Jesus.*

I had finally texted our children and told them the words we did not want to hear: *probably cancer.* But I couldn't help adding: *It may not be. We have to wait and see.*

Pondering

Have you ever noticed that your perception of an event is not the same as someone else's? Have you considered that their past may impact how they see things?

Could you identify with Justin's reaction—denial –"This can't be happening to us"? Why is it so hard for us to ask for prayers? What happens when we let someone see we are vulnerable and hurting?

Chapter 4

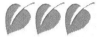

I Should Have Known

I am still confident of this: I will see the goodness of the Lord in the land of the living. Wait for the Lord; be strong and take heart and wait for the Lord. Psalm 27:13

January 19 began at 7 a.m. with a biopsy. Then the wait: Monday, Monday night, Tuesday, Tuesday evening, Wednesday, Wednesday evening . . . . We had just finished something for supper when the phone rang. "Can you get Wayne on an extension? I would like to talk to both of you." The doctor's tone was somber.

Wayne did not move as I ran for the extension.

"Go ahead, we're both listening."

"I got the results of the biopsy. . . . Not what we expected. . . . It is cancer . . . small cell, neuro-endocrine, stage 3, aggressive, in the lymph glands."

Silence. How do we respond to this? He hesitated, adding, "I'll make an appointment with the oncologist as soon as possible."

"Okay." We tried to breathe. Mind-bending, stomach-twisting fear attacked. We reached for each other and wept.

I knew the family was waiting for news, but it took almost an hour before I could write the text message. Reasons: the letters on my phone were a blur through my tears; I worried that they were putting our grandchildren to bed; I wanted to protect them from this earthquake a little longer; I did not want to admit life had changed, not like this; and I knew they would call, but we couldn't speak.

*****

I should have known. I should have known from a lifetime of walking in faith. But then again, a cancer diagnosis attacks the mind and the spirit. Thank God He understands and shows up through fractured prayers and sleepless nights. I should have known He would. I should have known He would use people to be His hands and heart to us. I should have trusted more, but He had to quiet my heart enough to see His care and refocus my thoughts. He drew us closer through His Word and prayer, and then used our children to minister to our brokenness. There would be other people in the months ahead, but He began with them. They love Him too. He showed up. They showed up. And what a difference it made. I should have known, but it was okay. I'm not strong. He is.

*****

Wednesday night we got the news. Friday morning Wayne was back in the hospital for a complete body scan to see how far the cancer had spread. I assured the kids we would be fine. They all have busy lives. But when we walked into the hospital lobby, two smiling men were there waiting. Jordan and Justin had taken off from work to sit and wait with me. Hour stretched into hour and despite my urging them to leave, they stayed. This became their habit. The seven: our two daughters, our two sons, our daughter-in-law, our sons-in-law, would consult and decide who would be there for many of the appointments that would fill the next months. I have tried to tell them, but I don't think they really know, how much that helped.

*****

I shouldn't have been surprised. God had been working in their lives for many years, maturing them. I remember one of the first times I made a decision to accept that fact. We were driving from Michigan to South Carolina for a vacation. It complicated the plan when Wayne had to work until midnight, so we had found a late flight for him. The boys (teenagers at the time) and I left on time to drive straight to Savannah and pick him up from the airport. Jordan had recently gotten his driver's license and did some of the driving which he enjoyed and gave me a break.

Somewhere near a large city we got stuck in traffic. After hours of crawling along I really needed a restroom. I told Jordan to pull off the highway even though I knew we were not in an ideal location. He found

16

a small restaurant, pulled over and parked. I told them to lock the doors and I would be right back. Before I could turn to close my door, both boys had jumped out and stood on each side of me. Ignoring my protests they said, "We'll come with you." It suddenly dawned on me that they had taken on the mantle of protectors, and it was time to embrace that.

All eyes from the counter people to the men sitting at the small lunch tables turned as we pushed the creaking door open. We smiled, and I asked if I might use their rest room. "No problem," the man behind the counter replied and nodded in the right direction. The boys, correction—young men of mine—slouched their six foot plus frames against the wall and waited. It was an epiphany for me. Our sons were becoming the men we had prayed they would be.

*****

Those men, our sons, sat with me as the time dragged on while Wayne was having the scan, far past the hour he should have been finished. Wayne had been called in shortly after we arrived in the waiting room at Metro Hospital. Later he told me the delay seemed to involve a computer glitch that would not read his hospital bracelet I.D. When he saw that the technician was getting frustrated, he told her, "I do have my Family Fare Grocery Card, if that will help." She laughed. Wayne has a knack for that.

Our kids would ask me how Dad and I fell in love. Wayne loves sports, especially golf, has a witty sense of humor, and a passion for music. Me, I love books. I taught English, piano lessons, wrote and led Bible studies and, I admit, I'm a bit on the serious side. Perhaps opposites attract, but it is more than that. First, I was simply drawn to his good looks, especially his smile. When he saw me in the hallways at school, his intense blue eyes lingered; he smiled; and I found myself grinning back. I loved that he could make me laugh, slow down, savor life, and not get so wound up about the next math test.

That's how it began, and it grew from attraction, to friendship, to love. That love deepened for me as I discovered he was a man of faith, a man of integrity, a man I could trust. The fact that he has continued to make me smile, and even laugh, has always enriched my love.

Once when the kids were in school and he had a day off, he agreed to help me get through my to-do list which included a trip to a big box store. I briskly walked up and down the aisles checking off each item on my list as I found it in the nearly empty store. Meanwhile, he was strolling through the aisles noting the variety of products offered and tuning his ear to the music playing.

My cart was full when I rejoined him. He grinned when he saw me, "Can I have this dance?" Finally, I stopped and listened. It was an old favorite from our first year of marriage. Glancing around and seeing no one, I accepted his offer, and we danced together to *Have You Ever Seen the Rain.*

I treasure that memory and thought it was unwitnessed until he told me much later, "When we were standing in the checkout lane and you ran for something, an employee came up to me and asked if we were the couple dancing in Aisle Seven. I admitted we were. He said, 'That was cool.'"

The kids loved that unpredictable side of their dad and remember when they were young, after a supper which included vegetables and fruit (a balanced diet—my thing), he had told them to get any bowl they wanted. When they asked, "For what?" he said, "Dessert of course!" They still love to recall the night they ate ice cream sundaes out of serving bowls, mixing bowls, and even a pan!

Pondering

How do you give yourself time to grieve and process disappointing news? What abilities do you see in your maturing children? Your adult children? Or other family members? How are they a part of the comfort God sends?

Why do we resist allowing our grown children the chance to nurture and care for us?

Chapter 5

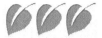

Unexpected Help

"Love the Lord your God . . . Love your neighbor as yourself" . . . . *"And who is my neighbor?"* In reply Jesus said: *"A man was going down from Jerusalem to Jericho when he fell into the hands of robbers."* Luke 10:27-29

Once when I found my five year old granddaughter crying, I lifted her onto my lap and asked her what was wrong. "My heart is black and blue it hurts so much." Her answer pierced me, painting a picture of her sadness.

An unexpected crisis can feel like getting your heart beaten up. It feels like *falling into the hands of robbers.* It steals your peace, your health, your security and leaves you feeling battered.

The initial diagnosis spurred me to push aside feelings and make battle plans. But as the days and weeks and months passed with the relentless demands of the disease, I could not ignore that my heart was black and blue from the struggle. Melancholy and depression threatened to move in and make a home in my mind and spirit. I went through stages of grief, anger, and sadness.

I even questioned God's love at times throwing my doubts, fears, and anger at Him. *Why are you letting this happen? Enough already. I know it's a test, but haven't we gone through enough tests—shattered dreams, financial losses, grading papers until I fell asleep with the pen sliding off the page leaving a trail of red ink? Life seems so much easier for lots of people. Give us a break!*

Pain strips us of subtle dishonesty and leaves raw emotions. I wanted to be strong for Wayne, for the family. But there were times when I was alone, especially in the hours before dawn, when my heart cried out to God in frustration and fear, weary of the struggle and sad. I felt like a reed crushed in the storm. Would God respond to my lack of faith, my anger, my self-pity?

Thank God His love depends on His character, not mine. The mustard seed of faith that made me draw near to Him brought His light into our dark places. At times I felt like Jacob wrestling through the night (Genesis 32:22-32). I would not let God go until He blessed me with some peace. Throughout our long journey, through my struggles, God was faithful. I learned to claim the promises like: *A bruised reed He will not break, and a smoldering wick He will not snuff out* (Isaiah 42:3). *And I have chosen you and have not rejected you. So do not fear, for I am with you; do not be dismayed, for I am your God. I will strengthen you and help you; I will uphold you with my righteous right hand* (Isaiah 41:9b-10).

One way He revealed His love and faithfulness was through a lesson we had to learn that was a key to resources God had provided for us. That key came in an old, familiar story told in the gospel of Luke.

Jesus was often tested by experts trying to make Him look foolish and discredit Him. These incidents are recorded in the Bible. Due to the amazing power of the *living Word* of God they can reveal timeless insights that speak to our deepest needs today. Luke 10:25-37 is one of the most frequently studied for just that reason. It teaches, among other things, an important lesson to people like me who suffer, but still want to be in control, still want to determine the plan.

In answer to the question, "What must I do to inherit eternal life?" Jesus told the interrogator: "Love the Lord your God with all your heart and with all your soul and with all your strength and with all your mind; and, Love your neighbor as yourself." The expert, probably looking for a loophole, or realizing he could not do that perfectly, asked, "Who is my neighbor?" That question generated the powerful story of the Good Samaritan.

Jesus said there was a man traveling from Jerusalem to Jericho, a very dangerous but frequently traveled road familiar to His listeners. Jews often traveled back and forth between these two cities. This traveler was jumped by robbers who not only stole his goods, they also beat him and left him near death by the side of the road.

Potential help arrived in the form of two distinguished Jews who came by and saw their fellow countryman lying there, helpless. Each of them thought of a reason not to stop. So the suffering victim remained. I imagine him coming to, barely able to see through swollen eyes, every part of his body aching, crying out in his spirit, *God, help me!*

Suddenly, he felt gentle hands cleaning his wounds, pouring oil on them, bandaging them. He heard quiet words of encouragement. Perhaps he thought, *Dad came. No, that's not his voice; he must have sent someone to find me, must be someone from town.* Can you imagine his shock when he realized his helper was no one he would have expected— a complete stranger, and a Samaritan (a group of people the Jews held in disdain)?

The Jewish traveler could not have been rescued by a kinder, more generous, godly person. What a pity it would have been if he had turned him away because it was not who he thought should have come!

Our journey was like that at times, help coming from unexpected sources. Margaret Feinberg in her wonderful book, *Fight Back with Joy*, writes eloquently of her battle with cancer and the blessings of people who poured oil on her wounded spirit. She also warns that sometimes it is not from the people you expect to be there.

I needed to learn that. I admit when I asked God for help, I expected certain people to show up in answer to that prayer. When they didn't, or told me it was too difficult to see Wayne so thin and unlike himself, my first reaction was hurt, even bitter disappointment. Not a good place to be emotionally. Like the seeds of anger, or envy, bitterness can take root and poison a heart.

There had to be a better response. Like the Jewish traveler, we were offered and learned to accept comfort from unexpected sources. I needed to trust my Father more and let go of control and expectations. I needed to make room for grace in all its amazing forms. His provision was so much more gracious than anything I could have imagined.

There were times our door bell would ring and an acquaintance we did not know very well would be standing on the front porch. It makes me smile now to think of the grace they brought when they stopped and said words to the effect, "I just felt a nudge to stop by and let you know our family is praying for you." Or "I made some cookies and thought I would bring some over and say hi." And then there were two neighbor men, Rob and Art, who stopped by and asked to see Wayne. They stood on the front porch and prayed over him, and then asked if he would like to take a walk. That was in the middle of heavy treatment, and they matched their steps to Wayne's slower ones. Grace, opening the door to grace.

And the people I had thought disappointed me? Sometimes I had to forgive; sometimes just realize that they showed up in other ways, ways God had guided them.

I learned to stop trying to direct the music of consolation and listen; I learned to recognize and be thankful for whispers of grace; to make room for the soothing oil of the unexpected blessing. I learned to entrust my black and blue heart to my Father's love and care more deeply.

I also needed to tune my heart to the nudges of the Holy Spirit to reach out to fellow travelers in need who crossed my path. My understanding of neighbors has grown. My awareness of God's provision is deeper.

Pondering

Have you wondered why painful trials come? How have you reacted? Can you recall a whisper of grace? —an unexpected offer of comfort?

Have you experienced the God-nudge to step out and help, even if you did not quite understand why?

Chapter 6

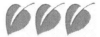

Grandkids, a Play, and a Hockey Game

Jesus said, "Let the little children come to me, and do not hinder them, for the kingdom of God belongs to such as these. I tell you the truth, anyone who will not receive the kingdom of God like a little child will never enter it." Luke 18:16-17

Stephanie, Paul, and their three girls, Grace, Aubrey, and Ashlyn, live two hours from our home. They had gotten the news Wednesday night. The phone calls and text messages had been flying back and forth, but sometimes, that just isn't enough. They came over for the weekend, something they would do many weekends in the months ahead.

The events of that weekend revealed God in unusual ways. He sent comfort and encouragement through His little children, a Good Samaritan, and a hockey game. It was the grandchildren who led the way. It began when the seventeen of us met together at Brad and Meredith's home on Saturday, just four days after the shattering news.

Our grandchildren—I thought distracted by the sheer delight they take in seeing each other and playing together—were dealing with the news in their own way, taking their cues from their parents. Just before supper they insisted we all come downstairs to Meredith's storage/laundry room. It includes a large, unfinished section which Meredith's girls had claimed as an Art Room. Two rows of folding chairs were lined up facing the washer and dryer; each one taped with a name tag. Papa was assigned the front and center seat.

Lauren, nine at the time, announced the production of the play they had written and were performing in honor of Papa. For the past hour they had been writing, staging, creating costumes, and practicing this masterpiece.

The opening scene revealed an adorable but spoiled Princess Ryan who was driving the maids crazy by throwing her clothes and toys everywhere. She treated the maids dreadfully. Their only friends were their brooms, which served double duties as sweepers and dance partners. In Scene Two the maids had had enough and planned to quit and run away, but first they warned the princess that her behavior was wrong. But then, tragedy struck. Queen Lauren was sick and needed help. In Scene Three, the princess turned to the maids for help. They changed their plans and came to the rescue. Princess Ryan transformed into a grateful and helpful child.

All the actors and actresses, ages five to ten, took deep bows to our appreciative laughter and applause, followed by a rush to pile on Papa's lap to tell him they loved him. Sometimes laughter and tears mingle.

Months later I asked them what they remembered about finding out Papa had cancer. Considering it was long ago in their lifetime, I was amazed at how vivid their memories were and how eager they were to share them. Sometimes I think adults believe that children are unaware and unable to handle the hard times life brings. I do not believe we help them when we leave them confused and tell them, "Don't worry about it." Saying those words doesn't release the fear from their hearts.

Being sensitive to their fears is a gift our children gave our grandchildren. Each set of parents sat down with their children to tell them "Papa has cancer." Their reactions reflected their ages and their personalities. Each child was encouraged to ask questions. Each one was given freedom to respond in ways that made them feel included in the fight. Interestingly, I know now, each child found a lot of comfort in their cousins and simply in being together.

Grace, our oldest grandchild, was ten at the time. She told me, *I knew something was wrong when we got home from school and mom was on the phone, crying. I took my sisters upstairs to play for a while until mom came and talked to us. I was sad and afraid for Papa. It made me understand how sad some of my friends at school felt because their grandparents had died.*

Lauren remembers: *It was a Thursday afternoon after school. Mom and Dad asked us to sit down at the table. They had some sad news to share. Papa has cancer. Friday at school wasn't prayer request day, but I told my teacher anyway, and we prayed for Papa.* Months later I met Lauren's teacher and found out Lauren and her classmates prayed for Papa week after week.

Aubrey, Grace's sister, eight years old when all this started, had her own reactions to what was happening. She told me *I think God let this happen to our family to prepare us to do something else.* She told me how sad she felt and when she went to school the next day her friends noticed, *because I wasn't bouncy and cheerful. My teacher noticed too and asked me what was wrong. When I told them, they were very kind to me and some of them even said they would pray for Papa. I worried that Papa would be in the hospital a lot, and we wouldn't see him.*

Hannah, who had just turned six, told me she worried that *Papa wouldn't be funny anymore.* Like Hannah, William was six, and worried *that he wouldn't be able to see Papa and do fun things like play baseball.*

They had seen sadness on their parents' faces and responded with prayers, love, and action.

After the play and supper God had another surprise waiting for us. Our sons had thought it would be fun to take their dad to a Griffins' hockey game that night. The Griffins are a professional team affiliated with the Detroit Red Wings, and very popular in town. Phone calls were made, a few last minute tickets were available, but the grandkids all wanted to go too.

Jordan left the room and came back with a grin on his face. "How would everyone like to go to the game? I just got a call from a friend who loaned us his suite. There's room for all of us." The grandkids didn't know what a suite was, but they were excited to be included. The adults knew what a suite was and the rare treat they were in for. Even 18 month old Andrew caught the excitement and began laughing.

I did not know this "good Samaritan" who had provided for us, but I thanked God for him.

The blustery cold night didn't keep any hardy Griffins fans from making the trek to Van Andel Arena. We piled into three vehicles, followed each other downtown, and then scattered as we searched for parking, regrouping in the crowded lobby. The little ones were giddy with the crowds and palpable excitement that filled the lobby. Jordan led the way up the stairs, found the suite number, and was greeted by a waitress awaiting our arrival.

The suite included an interior room with a table, comfortable chairs, a television, and even a private bathroom. The smell of fresh popcorn filled the air and bowls of it and cans of soft drinks seemed to magically appear. The exterior section was visible and accessible through the glass-sided wall and included two rows of seats on a balcony overlooking the crowded arena. A glass door could be left open or closed, which proved helpful especially when Andrew needed a break from the noise.

The arena camera began searching the crowd for excited fans dancing to the pounding music. It wasn't long before they found seven children dancing with delight on the balcony. Seeing themselves on the large overhead screen in the middle of the arena put them over the moon.

"Grandma, I've never been in a suite in my whole life. And I am 10! It's awesome!" Grace bubbled.

"And I'm a grandma, and I've never been in a suite either! It is awesome!" We grinned at each other.

The game began and my six year old grandson William climbed on my lap. He had never been to a hockey game before, but he had begun to develop a passion for sports. Along with that passion was a need to understand the intricacies of each game he saw or played. So the questions began. How many players were there? What were the players' positions? I was quickly in over my head.

My son-in-law Paul was sitting behind us. I made the mistake of mentioning that Uncle Paul played hockey every Friday night. Mistake because I was really enjoying my time with William, and once I said that he slipped off my lap and sidled up to Uncle Paul with a question, "Do you really play hockey?" Soon he was settled on Paul's lap. For the next hour Paul patiently answered every question and described the game, the equipment, and the action, feeding the curiosity of a little boy who would make hockey his favorite sport, at least until springtime.

What I remember about that night is seeing the smiles, hearing the laughter, feeling the love of my family, and experiencing incredible gratitude that God could infuse a painful week with joy. I would go back to these memories in the months ahead, when I needed reminders that God is faithful.

Pondering

Children have their own fears. How do they express them? Different ages react differently. What differences have you noticed? How do children offer comfort in their own creative ways?

How do you leave room for laughter? Are you flexible? "Out-of-the-mouth-of-babes" moments are precious. Can you recall some?

Chapter 7

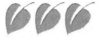

"Strange Thankfulness"

The Lord is my Shepherd . . . even though I walk through the valley of the shadow of death... Psalm 23:1, 4

I knew our children were going through their own struggles as the awareness of what we were facing settled in. I have asked each one what they remember. Some can only answer with tears in their eyes as they relive those days; some have been able to articulate in writing.

Brad wrote to me: *When we got the results it was like a punch in the gut. I knew I shouldn't google it, but right away I did, and what I saw was very scary. Survival rates were low. Most of these types of cancer were tied to the lungs and had awful results. This was a dark place that we'd never been. Our "go to" lines and verses about our faith didn't seem good enough. We knew we had to depend on God, but in a much different way than our previous struggles in life. This was one that none of us could do on our own and we truly needed His strength and peace.*

There are so many emotions, it is hard to tell where they are coming from. I was sad for you (Mom) and Dad because of how much you love each other. I thought about if it were me finding this out about Meredith how I would feel. I was sad for Meredith and the thought of her losing her dad. I was sad for myself because of how much I love Dad. I knew I shouldn't go to the thought of loss, but that's where I went. My saddest thought might have been thinking that my son might not know his papa and get to have the impactful relationship with Dad that I've had. Dad has a number of qualities that I don't have and that I won't ever have. His genuine love for life and thankfulness for each day overflows in the way he lives and I want Andrew to taste that. Dad is different than most Christian role models that I knew growing up, and I'm a better person because of him.

The thought of Andrew not learning from and enjoying this joy for life was heartbreaking. I wondered if I'd ever be able to golf with Drew and Dad.

When it came time to tell the girls, I was shocked that I couldn't even talk. I couldn't bring myself to talk about it, which was surprising. Typically, Meredith is the crier and I'm the level-headed, consistent one. But on this day, she had to tell them. I was a mess. Somehow she could talk at that moment and stay calm. There were many other times that she couldn't talk about it, but at that moment, God gave her the words and the composure to tell them that God would take care of us. I was able to talk with them later and answer their questions, but it took me a while. I wanted our girls to know that God was in control. I wanted them to know that we didn't know what that meant, but that He promised to uphold us no matter what. I wanted to model a faith that I wasn't even sure I had at that moment.

As the news settled in I struggled with how to apply my faith to this fight. I know that God has a plan and that He will care for us. I know that life on earth is a vapor and that our eternal home isn't this one. But that didn't change how sad we were. The reality is that because we love Dad so much and because we have been so blessed to have three generations of loving family, this was an even more difficult time. It humbles me to think about those who can't share their darkest times with the people around them. I thought about how lonely this journey could be for those who don't have what we have. It was a reminder to me that God didn't create us to do this alone. He commands us to cast all our burdens on Him. Maybe I've not done the best job of this because I have such an amazing support system. Maybe I've tried to do too much on my own or with the help of others rather than with God by my side. These trials brought these thoughts to my head because we couldn't do this without Him.

Even throughout that pain, Meredith and I realized how blessed we were to have a father whose loss could produce such pain. There was a strange thankfulness that came with the heartache. If this life is a vapor, how awesome that we get to go through our trials in Christian community. How awesome that my kids get to witness generations relying on God even in the face of death.

Jordan was also able to write his thoughts. He is a problem solver and immediately needed facts: *I made the rookie mistake of googling terms like small cell, carcinoma, and neuroendocrine. If you go looking for bad news, the internet will deliver by the truckload. Cursory research on survival rates and treatment plans brought little comfort. The scariest thing was the possibility that the cancer had metastasized and we would not have even the shot at treatment options. I remember hoping and praying that there was at least a shot. I knew we had no idea. I went right to playing out the worst-case scenarios, most notably my kids would grow up without one of their grandfathers. I was about William's age when my grandfather died, and I tried to remember what I felt and what I understood.*

Jordan was seven years old when my dad, Neil Greydanus, died. The call came in the middle of the night from Florida. "Dad's gone." I doubled over with the physical pain of his loss. I had flown down to see Mom and Dad five weeks earlier, by myself, knowing Dad's heart was struggling. Dad and I had played golf together, just nine holes, taking our time. Then we stopped to pick up a Valentine's Day card for Mom. We laughed when we discovered the card division marked "Religious Wife" knowing we would find the perfect card in that section. We stopped for Dad's hearing test. Mom had been complaining that dad wasn't listening. His hearing was fine. He promised he would do better with his "selective hearing." Precious intimate moments with the man who believed in me when I didn't believe in myself, the father who loved me, the grandfather who treasured my children, his grandchildren.

The funeral was held in New Jersey. As soon as we arrived at the funeral home Jordan and Justin (5 years old) ran ahead of us to the casket and Jordan grabbed his grandpa's hand. He recoiled in shock. He turned to me, "Mom, Grandpa's cold. What's wrong?" Every trip to New Jersey had included hours with his grandpa laughing and playing cars on the floor. He had felt the warmth of his grandpa's hand holding his when they walked together. Jordan had never seen death before. How could I comfort him when I was aching with grief?

"Grandpa's in Heaven. He has a new body. He's feeling great today."

"But he's cold."

God help, how do I explain this?

"Do you remember when I cut your fingernails and toenails? What do we do with the little pieces?"

"You throw them away."

"Do you miss them?"

His expression let me know that was ridiculous. "No way."

"Do you miss the hair that gets thrown away when you get a haircut?"

"No." His expression began to change and my heartache eased.

"This body is like your nail clips and hair snips. Grandpa doesn't need it. We'll miss him, but we'll see him again when we get to Heaven."

Perhaps Jordan would have to use that insight with William.

Leah has a sensitive, loving spirit which is so evident in these words she wrote to me: *I wouldn't say I responded to the "type" of cancer as much as the fact that it was indeed cancer. I had zero clue what kind of cancer that was. I remember trying to put myself in Jordan's shoes as all the texts were coming in. What if this were my dad? How would I want to feel supported and loved at this time? I tried not to say too much or too little . . . lots of hugs and "I am so sorry, honey" and quiet prayers as the news settled in for us both. Being "one-step" removed, I wanted to make sure and support the family as a whole by being there for my husband. I knew he would want to step up and be involved on many levels and I wanted to make it ok for him to do whatever he felt he needed to do for you and Dad.*

Definitely there were more fears as we searched on line for information. It seemed like this type of cancer could mean a lot of different things. The weeks of waiting to hear if the cancer had spread and what the plan would be were tough. My most vivid memory is lying in bed with William one night as he fell asleep. I hadn't cried much yet about the whole thing. On this night I laid in bed with him and the thought struck me, "What if William isn't going to get to grow up with his papa? --the man he shares a name with and is supposed to secretly give him his first beer? Papa is supposed to give William all the great advice he won't listen to us for . . . and so on and so on . . . ." Finally the tears silently flowed that night.

Each family member was processing the news. I watched our daughters, Stephanie and Meredith. I know how much they love their dad and saw the ache in their eyes. Yet, I saw something else as well, courage. They swallowed their pain to be strong for their children; strong for us, their parents. They have such tender, nurturing spirits that it wasn't a surprise to us when they became social workers.

I still remember when they were teenagers, and we worked together for months to raise funds to go on a mission trip to Albania. I had promised to help them go, but they insisted the three of us should go together. I doubted that we could financially manage that. Their faith was unwavering. It took a sermon to convince me.

"Has God asked you to do something big? Are you afraid that it's impossible?" Those were the opening questions. I flinched when I heard them. The message was based on Joshua 2. God told Joshua to conquer Canaan and begin with one of the strongest, most fortified cities, Jericho.

"Be like this God-dependent believer, Joshua," the pastor encouraged us. "Wait for God's vision; Walk in Obedience; and Watch what God will do. He will take down the walls."

Four months later I watched my two girls as together we taught, played with, and embraced the orphans in Tirana, Albania. With them, I fell in love with the people and the country. The last day as we said good-bye, the little ones they had loved for Jesus clung to the girls. Both of them untangled little arms, gently separated themselves, smiled, and slipped out of the gates. Out of sight, they sobbed. Their hearts forever impacted by the needs of this world.

Pondering

When bad news comes, what helps? What doesn't help? Have you noticed that other people react and process bad news differently? It can be difficult letting family, friends, or the church know what is happening. Why is that? What are the benefits?

Is there room for gratitude? Did Brad's feelings of "strange thankfulness" that came with the heartache make sense to you?

Chapter 8

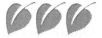

Faith Fortified

O Lord, hear my prayer, listen to my cry for mercy; in your faithfulness and righteousness come to my relief. Psalm 143:1

Sunday morning, in that semi-awake moment before full consciousness, I reveled in the memories of the play, the hockey game, the family. Within seconds I felt my chest tighten as I also remembered why we were together, and that in less than twenty-four hours Wayne would be at St. Mary's Hospital in surgery for the stent. Our war against cancer was just beginning.

A cloud of despair began to suck the delight of the memories, replacing it with fear of the future. No! I would not go there. I rolled over, placed my hand on Wayne's shoulder, and prayed: *Bless the Lord oh my soul, and all that is within me, bless His holy name. Bless the Lord, oh my soul, and forget not all His benefits—who forgives all our iniquities and heals all our disease*s. God brought to mind verses from Psalm 103, and over and over again, they would be my first prayer of the morning.

Like many people who have suffered and are suffering, I turn to prayer and the book of Psalms which give voice to the anguish of the soul, the cry of the heart, and the hope believers find in God.

I still don't understand why God chooses to act through prayer. I'm never sure how or when He will answer, but I do know He always does. Sometimes God answers, "Yes," immediately, sometimes He says, "No," and sometimes His answer comes to me when I am ready to listen.

Two memories come to mind among many when I think of how God has answered my prayers. The first came back after one of my grandchildren told me, "Grandma, I can pray anywhere, even with my eyes open! God hears me!" Her faith reminded me of one such prayer I lifted as I walked down a crowded middle school hallway years ago. I had just left the school office. The secretary had commented while she handed me my keys and the substitute teaching plans, "Just call the office when it gets too wild. The principal is down at that room a couple times a day."

Yikes, what a warning! Searching for the room I prayed with eyes open, *Help Father. Give me an idea. Maybe this substitute teaching idea wasn't such a good one. I want out! Help me help these students.*

I stood near the door and watched the class jostle each other as they made their way in, completely ignoring me. Suddenly, I knew what to do. Watching for another moment I chose the loudest student surrounded by the most followers. I caught his attention and motioned for him to come to the front of the room. He towered over me. "Good morning. I'm obviously the substitute teacher today. And you are obviously the class leader."

He leaned closer to hear me over the chatter in the room, looking surprised, but pleased. "I would like to work with you, and if you help me, I promise to teach you something that could change your future."

"What do you want me to do?"

"Have everyone sit down and be quiet."

Each hour I found the leader, and each hour we completed the assignment with little trouble. The last few minutes of the class I fulfilled my promise and taught them something I had learned in my business experiences. First, I asked them to take out a paper. "You'll want to keep this paper somewhere special for years to come." They looked at me obviously wondering what could be that important. "It's important because it will hold your hopes and dreams and how you will get there."

"Ready? Okay. Write your name, today's date, and your current age. Skip a line and write *Ten Years from Now*. In a sentence or two write what you hope to be doing and where you will be. You'll be 24 or 25." I gave them a minute to write. "Now skip a line and write *Five Years from Now* and tell yourself where you will be then and what you hope to be doing."

After a moment, "Now you are doing what only the top achievers in life do: You are setting goals. You need one final piece. Skip a line and write *To get there I must . . . .* The decisions you make today shape your tomorrows. What are you willing to do to make your dreams come true? Write down at least three actions you will take. Maybe it's studying 15 minutes a day without distractions. Maybe it's going to bed on time. Only you know what you need. Want to be a success? Make a plan." Each class period ended with the gentle scratching of pencils and thoughtful silence.

God answered that eyes-open prayer immediately with a creative idea. But other times I prayed for years, persistently, before I heard the answer.

"Mom, don't you hear Justin?! He's crying." Nine year old Stephanie was exasperated with me. Horrified, I ran upstairs to find two year old Justin standing in his crib wailing for me with outstretched arms.

How long had he been calling, waiting? I scooped him up and pressed his tear-stained face to my shoulder as I confronted the truth of my hearing loss. *Really! Really God!* Anger and grief replaced the denial of my increasing disability. I was only in my mid-30s, but I was losing my hearing.

I confided in a friend who said it could just be ear wax. *Please God, let it be that.* The answer was "No." It was hearing loss that required a hearing aid. I begged God to restore my hearing even while I tried to adjust to my new reality.

My hair had been cut short. I let it grow to hide the embarrassment I felt, thinking everyone who saw me first saw that thing in my ear. For years I carried a festering resentment that God had refused to fix my problem.

Stephanie and I were shopping for her high school prom dress when I met a stranger God used to answer my prayers—not the answer I wanted, but the answer I needed.

"Can I help you? Let me take that to the dressing room for you." Her smile enhanced her lovely young face. She tucked her long brown hair behind her ears as she handed Steph another dress to try. That's when I noticed her hearing aid.

"You wear a hearing aid," I blurted, immediately feeling foolish. Trying to explain I added, "I wear one."

"Oh, I have two, and I thank God every day for them. Without them I couldn't hear my kids or my customers." Her smile was radiant.

Something in me snapped. Gratitude? Had I ever said thank you for what I considered my burden? That day, after patiently listening to my complaining prayers for years, God finally got through to me. I still wear hearing aids, two now in fact. Every morning they are the first things I put on and the last things I remove every night. Every day I thank Him for this gift of hearing.

How would God answer my desperate prayers for Wayne and our family? He did not make me wait long for one of His answers that

Sunday morning when despair threatened to take up residence in my spirit. He had tuned my heart to listen more clearly.

As we hurried into church that Sunday morning with Stephanie, Paul and the girls, we were surprised to see Jordan, Leah, Meredith, Brad, Justin and the grandkids saving seats. Justin goes to Calvary. In fact, he was the one who had encouraged us to try Calvary Church when he was in junior high and attended with a friend. But the others had their own home churches.

They had decided to come and worship together. The song we sang that morning was one we had not sung very often, but it became our theme song. The words had never soaked in like they did that morning. But then, I had never needed them so much. They spoke of our faithful God, our Heavenly Father who fights for us (Joshua 23:10). I could only mouth them as I tried to hide my tears.

Thank you Chris Tomlin for giving us this message in your beautiful song "Whom Shall I Fear?" It's so comforting to know that "the God of angel armies is always by our side."

Pondering

Fear is powerful. How do you handle fear? How do you fortify faith?

Can you recall a sudden answer to prayer? —or a prayer that was answered after a season?

Do you have a Psalm and a song that plays in your mind, reminding you of God's faithfulness and love? Feel free to adopt the ones God gave us.

Chapter 9

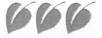

Counsel

. . . the wise listen to advice. Proverbs 12:15b

On the surface it looked like many other Sundays: church, Sunday dinner, family time. But the intruder in the room cast a shadow. As soon as the grandchildren went downstairs to play, even before the dishes were done, the questions and discussion turned to battle plans. Had we considered a second opinion? Yes. Where? I had been online looking for the best options; so had the family.

All of my life I have been keenly aware of the destructive nature of cancer. One of my brothers, a beautiful, precocious kindergartener who loved to share the Bible stories he learned in school, was diagnosed with leukemia and died a few weeks later at the age of five and a half. I never met him; I was born seven months later, but I knew him from my mom and dad's stories, old pictures, grainy movies, and the tears that sometimes filled my mother's eyes.

My grandmother died of colon cancer when I was a teenager. My mother was diagnosed with colon cancer several years after my dad died. She was 83, living alone in their beloved Florida home. The cancer was caught early. After her surgery I flew down to care for her for a week. She loved Bible study. I treasure the memories of talking with her about her most passionate interest—her Savior. She lived on her own for ten more years. My brother Stu and his family lived down the street and brought both protection and fun into her life.

Finally, at 93 she needed assisted living. She came to Michigan where I found Sunset Manor, a place of kindness and Christian care. I remember the first night she spent there. She hugged me and smiled, "Take good care of yourself. You belong to me," her favorite parting words. I tucked her in and made it to the quiet hallway before my eyes overflowed. I felt like a traitor even though I knew I could not keep up the 24/7 care I had given her for the last five weeks. As I leaned against the wall by her door, I seriously considered packing her up and taking her home.

"Oh, honey. She is going to be happy here." An aide had seen me and put her hand on my shoulder. "You know we don't work here because we need a job. This is a calling. Jesus called me here."

Mom lived there for two years and loved it. When she moved to Brookcrest for nursing care she got a reputation for her smiles, quiet thank-yous, and her peaceful spirit. Her life verse stayed with her even as her memory faded: *You will keep in perfect peace those whose minds are steadfast, because they trust in you.* Isaiah 26:3 She trusted, and He was faithful. Knowing her life on earth was coming to an end, I called other family members to come and say good-bye. Mom quietly smiled at each one and mouthed, "I love you." She passed away one week before her 97th birthday. She left me a legacy of faith that would be tested as hers was. Was mine as strong?

Our family tree is riddled with a variety of cancer diagnoses. For years I have wondered when, not if, I too will wage war with this enemy. Articles and internet sites about cancer prevention, antioxidants, and cancer treatment often catch my attention. The amount of information available is staggering. How to sift through it and find the answers we needed? How quickly the awareness of cancer became an intense personal scramble to learn everything we could, as fast as we could.

Wayne's family had experienced few cancers until recently. He had been the picture of health for most of our marriage. His diagnosis shocked both of us, and I learned that just adjusting to the news can suck up most of one's emotional and mental resources.

We needed wisdom to make the decisions that lay before us. Simply admitting we did not have all the answers was a relief and opened the door to help. One lesson we learned years earlier from our pastor came to mind.

We joined Calvary Church in large part because of the dynamic, Bible-based preaching of Ed Dobson. His passion for Jesus, knowledge of scripture, humor, and practical applications made each Sunday service a feast we carried home with us. When he was diagnosed with ALS, (amyotrophic lateral sclerosis) better known as Lou Gehrig's disease, in the prime of his life, his ministry to us did not end.

Encouraged by Ed to dig into the scriptures ourselves, I often carried my Bible to church in order to take notes in the margins. One of those notes lit up when we faced our crisis years after Ed had to relinquish his responsibilities at church. I wrote it the year after he had retired and returned to preach for one morning. He said that before he asked for healing, he asked for wisdom. Many people offered him advice and options. He asked God to give him wisdom: who to listen to, what to do, where to go. He reminded us that James 1:5-6 was a promise we could claim: *If any of you lacks wisdom, you should ask God, who gives generously to all without finding fault, and it will be given to you. But when you ask, you must believe and not doubt.* This would not be the last time God used Ed Dobson to bless us. More about that later.

So we prayed as a family, pooled our information, made lists, and considered which of the many choices we should pursue. Everyone agreed we should contact Mayo Clinic in Rochester, Minnesota. But how soon would we get an appointment? A growing sense of urgency spurred us to hurry. Every test had been quickly followed up by another. We had been urged not to miss one or delay treatment.

As the afternoon drew to a close and it was time for everyone to leave, there was one more discussion they wanted to have. They wanted to decide who would go with us to the first oncologist's appointment in a few days. Wayne and I assured them we would be fine and would text all of them about any important information we received.

I must confess wiser heads prevailed. Wiser for two reasons. The first is related to the reality of stress and its impact on the brain and critical thinking. Walking into Lemmen-Holton Cancer Pavilion (or any cancer clinic, I imagine) for the first time after receiving the diagnosis generates another level of stress as we are confronted with this reality: This is real, and it is going to be a long battle. Stress can interfere with the ability to remember what we were going to ask and what we needed to remember about the new information and details.

We agreed there would be stress, so I found a green notebook that became our constant companion for the next year. Each time we had an appointment I dated a page, named the doctor, and wrote questions we had as well as questions our children had thought of. I left some space between each question and wrote the answers we received. Meredith reminded me that it would be hard to listen and write everything down the first time. So we agreed she should come and be the recording secretary. Jordan also wanted to come to ask follow-up questions. Stephanie and Paul had to get their children back home for school, and Justin agreed to go to work. Meredith and Jordan promised on-going text messages. They all agreed to this plan, and, finally, so did we.

That leads to the second reason it was wise to accept their help and welcome their participation. Besides the fact that we needed them, they needed to be engaged. They were emotionally as well as intellectually involved with their dad's cancer. It comforted them to be with us, and it certainly comforted us to have them. They had insights we might have missed if we had resisted their help and refused to listen.

Pondering and a Game Plan

How do you make decisions? Prayer? People? Investigation? Who are some of the people you invite to share their thoughts? It might be family, or it might be a friend, church member, or someone you met as your journey began. Don't go it alone. Pray for companions to walk with you. It is hard to recognize our own limitations and the impact stress can have. Give some thought to what helps when people are stressed.

Do you have some way to keep track of the questions, answers, appointments, doctors' names, and plethora of information you will receive? (See Lessons Learned at the end of the book for our plan.)

Chapter 10

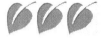

Tears

Those who sow with tears will reap with songs of joy. Psalm 126:5

As the weekend drew to a close and the family packed up to go home, I felt the wave of anxiety that had been held back sweeping over me. *God, please help me be strong. No tears until their car doors shut.* Perhaps it was motivated by pride. Whatever the reason, God let the tears leak past my defenses.

Role reversal is never easy. The embrace of my children offering their strong shoulders breached the dam of my tear-control. Still, I had to hide the tears from our grandchildren, and I did from all of them, except from the tender, persistent gaze of Aubrey who would not take her eyes away. She was only eight years old, but she did not turn away from adult pain. She lingered, hugged me again, and then ran downstairs although all the luggage was already in the car.

We found it later, after everyone had left. It is what she decided she could do, and did do, every time she came for a weekend. Sometimes she left them in our bedroom; sometimes downstairs on the table used for their art projects. What she left us were treasures: letters of her love and prayers written in crayon or markers in scrawling, third grade script.

Tears and being sensitive to the needs of others reminds me of one of our best family stories.

Two and a half years before our cancer journey began, Meredith and Brad embarked on a personal journey that we as a family willingly joined. On July 3 they were playing golf together when Meredith's cell phone rang. They were playing only nine holes, and had left their two daughters with Brad's parents, so the cell phone was turned on. How thankful they were that it was.

"Hello, Meredith. A baby boy was born yesterday. He is in the hospital and needs a foster home. Are you willing to take him, and can you pick him up tomorrow morning? Please let us know in the next fifteen minutes."

Twelve months earlier Meredith had felt strongly led to become a foster family. Brad soon joined her in the conviction that God was calling them to be foster parents. Together they enrolled in the necessary classes and were licensed. They were committed to love and care for a new baby who could stay for three days, three months, a year, or maybe forever.

Their willingness to risk the emotional pain of surrendering a baby I knew they would treasure took my breath away. Only their rock-solid belief that God was in this gave them the courage to prepare a nursery and see what God had planned.

Meredith wrote about these experiences: *February 2013, we shared our calling with Lauren and Hannah. Could they be foster sisters to a baby and help take care of him as long or short as God asked us to? They were instantly onboard wanting to know "When will he come?" But we had no answer, only faith in God's perfect timing. Like Noah building an ark, without a rain cloud in sight, we faithfully set up a crib and prayed for this baby and his birthparents. We filled out paperwork and prayed. Asked friends and bosses for references. We went to church, prayed, cried tears that meant God-at-work, and prepared our home and hearts.*

We can testify to James 4 where it says "Draw near to God and He will draw near to you." We asked for His presence and God . . . Showed Up. He was ever-present, opening doors like a new van, a new house, a new job, encouragement from friends and family, a care group with adoptive parents, and one of my favorites, winning WCSG's radio contest for housecleaning!

Our foster care license was completed June 2013. MaryJo our licensor, explained that once we got a call on a child needing placement, we would have 15 minutes to decide. My mind raced. Would we even be together? How do we know what to say?

Meredith received her answer through a song by Shirley Caesar: *That Sunday we sang "Yes, Lord, Yes." In my heart I said yes to His will and His way, to trust Him and obey Him with my whole heart. I felt my fears calm, and I had an answer. We would answer yes.*

Their daughters, Lauren and Hannah, had willingly moved into one bedroom together to make room. After the fresh paint had dried, the crib set up, and the changing table prepared, the girls asked every day, "Do you think the baby is coming today?"

Months rolled by and we as grandparents, Brad's folks and us, talked and prayed about the precious little one who was being "fearfully and wonderfully knit together in his mother's womb" (Psalm 139:13-14). Would he be part of the family for a short time, or a lifetime?

Some memories are permanent pictures in my mind. One of them is Meredith and Brad coming in to join us for the Fourth of July celebration holding a tiny bundle in a blue blanket. Hannah and Lauren had stayed with us while their parents went to the hospital. A pair of brown eyes and a pair of blue eyes shimmered with excitement as both girls reached out to hold their new foster brother.

There seemed to be a gentle breeze that passed over us as we circled the new family unit. To me, it was Holy-Spirit-blessings infusing the family with love for this little stranger who went from stranger to beloved in a fraction of a moment. He wrapped his hand around our fingers and our hearts.

Meredith was determined to give this little one the most loving welcome to life that she could. She used a baby wrap carrier to carry him on her chest so he could feel her heart beat, hear her voice, and be enfolded in her love. Oh, there was bonding.

That deep love from both Brad and Meredith helped them get through the challenging year which followed. Their calendar became filled with countless appointments including supervised birth parent visits, social worker visits, lawyer visits, court dates, and doctor appointments for checkups and breathing problems that plagued the baby. They invested deeply even while Meredith worked two part-time jobs. Aunt Beth babysat while Meredith worked, and she poured more love into him. As Meredith put it, "She is a gift to us!"

Meredith recalls, *And God was there. Helping us live in the reality of loving a baby we might not keep. Loving his birth parents and being loved by family and friends. We were tired and overwhelmed, but our hearts were full. I kept in mind the quote: "Outside the will of God, there's nothing I want. Inside the will of God, there's nothing I fear."*

Lauren used to ask me, "Grandma, do you think there's a 40 percent or 50 percent chance 'D' (his nickname) will become my forever brother and not my foster brother?" She was good at math and tried to calculate the future, increasing the numbers as the months passed.

Ten months after his arrival there was another court date, this one permanently etched in Brad and Meredith's memories. They had worked hard to build a relationship with the birth parents, to encourage them, sitting by them at court hearings. (Later the social worker commented,

"That rarely happens.") They assured them that they were on the same team. They loved the same baby boy and wanted what was best for him. These young parents loved their son, but finally they admitted they could not care for him.

In May, the birthparents made the difficult and loving decision to relinquish their rights. Outside the courtroom doors love trickled from overflowing eyes, and they asked us to adopt him. It was a holy moment. We thanked them for choosing life! We honor and remember them.

It would be months before Brad and Meredith could legally answer that question. The law had requirements that had to be met. One of the most important took the longest: relatives had to be found and contacted. Were they willing and able to adopt this baby boy?

Lauren would calculate, "I think it's 70 percent now, Grandma." I would watch her and Hannah play with him and see their longing. He was woven into the fabric of Meredith and Brad's family unit and our extended family. Hearts would be torn if he had to go.

Fourteen months after that first cell phone call on the golf course, another life-changing call was received from the court: "Are you willing to adopt your foster son?"

The court room was full on October 8, 2014 with family, friends, social workers, and a lawyer who had come to witness and bless the formal adoption day of the newest member of the family, Andrew, now 100 percent Lauren and Hannah's forever brother.

Stephanie had taken her girls out of school and driven two hours to the court house to join us. The night before she had seen Aubrey pacing around her bedroom and heard her talking to herself. She stopped in the hall to listen to a passionate plea to the judge to allow Aunt Meredith and Uncle Brad to adopt Andrew. There seemed to be a lingering fear that the odds might only be 95 percent. She wanted to do her part if she were called to testify to push it to 100 percent.

Judge G presided over the courtroom as we all sat quietly, except for fifteen month old Andrew, dressed in a white shirt, vest, and red tie matching his dad's. He was taking great delight in toddling around smiling. He seemed to sense the joy of the day. The judge obviously enjoyed special days like this and invited all present to share a comment about why they had come. Much to our surprise the cousins all stood up to welcome their new cousin and assure the judge that they would love Andrew, and he would have a great home.

Unbidden, tears filled my eyes. Aubrey was sitting next to me, watching. Before I could assure her, "I'm fine," she whispered, "Sometimes happiness leaks out of your eyes, Grandma."

Pondering

Have you been called to do something bold and risky? How did you help your family through the journey?

Have you experienced tears of sorrow, healing tears, tears of joy? Do you let yourself cry? Are tears a gift we need in this life? Do you believe that God will wipe away every one?

Chapter 11

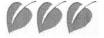

Thorns

I was given a thorn in my flesh. . . . But He said to me, "My grace is sufficient for you, for my power is made perfect in weakness."
II Corinthians 12:7, 9

The alarm was set for 5 a.m. on Monday. We didn't need it. Although we had both slept a few hours, we were up in plenty of time to make Wayne's 6 a.m. appointment at St. Mary's Hospital. It would result in an irritation that would aggravate him endlessly in the months ahead. The procedure would address the problem of the kidney that was shutting down. Inflammation from the cancer required a stent to be inserted that would allow the kidney to function.

As we stood in the back hall, ready to leave after collecting the green notebook, the three-ring binder with medical information, and a book that simply ended up lying on my lap; I put my arms around Wayne, felt the stifled sob, and prayed, "God, go with us. We need you."

We were in the waiting room for just a few minutes before a nurse called Wayne in to prep for the surgery. She gave me a number that would track Wayne's location and progress throughout the morning. It soon appeared with a dozen more on a large digital screen hanging on the wall. Thirty minutes later I joined him in the small prep cubicle dominated by a hospital bed. His blue eyes stood out in the dull white of the bed clothes and hospital gown; a smile played across his face when he saw me. A needle emerged from his right arm with a tube connected to an IV. Sitting on his left side, I could hold his hand. I just wanted to say, "Come on, let's get out of here."

Part of the cancer journey involves waiting: in hallways decorated with soothing art work; in waiting rooms of neatly lined-up chairs with fish tanks to lower blood pressure and magazines to offer a small mind-numbing distraction; in prep rooms with blinking lights reading blood pressure, heart rate, and announcing call buttons; in exam rooms furnished with computer screens which doctors' eyes search to study the patient seated across from them. Somehow minutes are longer when we sit there; communication is best done with the touch of a hand; and focused thoughts are fragmented with the concerns of the moment.

Those hours spent waiting deepened my understanding of the comfort in God's whisper, *Be still . . . Be still . . . Be still and know that I am God* (Psalm 46:10). My hands and tool box were empty. I had nothing to offer to fix the problem. The prickling pain in my heart demanded relief. It came through His words, *Be still and know*. What I came to know in the quietness of waiting was the intimate reality of His presence. Nothing soothed my anxieties compared to keeping my eyes on Jesus. So the protracted moments passed, and sometimes He sent relief in the form of His people.

That morning He sent two unexpected visitors and one I had specifically told not to come. Each one brought a blessing. The first was waiting for us, seated at a small table near the receptionist's desk. I did not recognize him, but after Wayne gave his name to the receptionist, and before he was called into the prep room, this white-haired gentleman slowly stood up and approached us. He told us he was from Calvary Church and had gotten word via the prayer chain that we would be here this morning. He wondered if he might pray with us for a moment. A stranger really, he had never met us before, and we did not know him. But somehow, in those few moments, he was our brother and reminded us God was with us. Then he left. I hope he reads this and knows how much that visit meant.

An hour later, as we waited in the curtained cubicle for Wayne's call to the operating room, a nurse stopped in, "Can Kevin come to see you?" She stepped aside so we could see the familiar face of our nephew. A St. Mary's work I.D. hung on his chest, but this visit wasn't official; it was personal. He had come in early just to offer his support. He liked to come over and fish on our small lake. He was good at fly fishing and easy banter. Distracted by talk of ice fishing and stories of past big ones, we both let our minds escape our current incarceration.

Our final visitor that morning had been clearly told not to come for her own sake. Her mornings were busy enough without a visit to us added to the schedule. But, as usual, when she did show up, we were glad to see her. Brad had delayed going to work to get Hannah and

Lauren off to school, and Meredith had bundled Andrew off to Aunt Beth's so she could make an early trek to the hospital. She arrived in time to help me wait out the surgery and hear what the doctor had to say.

Each of these visitors reminded me of how Jesus *puts on skin* through his people. Each one felt nudged by God to do something, and although inconvenienced, they responded with obedience and blessed us.

The number on the digital board flashed and informed me Wayne was in recovery. The receptionist told me to go to a small conference room where the doctor would meet me and explain the outcome of surgery. Meredith came with me. The doctor swept in wearing his surgical greens.

"Went well . . . kidney is functioning again. Wayne should be alert soon."

Relief as I listened to the report and instructions, but also a nagging question: "Are there any side effects or problems associated with this?"

His answer prepared me for what Wayne would experience, but not for how exasperating it would be for Wayne, or how it would impact routine activities.

"There might be some pressure on the bladder especially when he moves, but he should continue to drink a lot of water and lemonade."

For Wayne, just the movements required by daily routine meant pressure and prickling irritations. Some things you just don't want to think about all the time. Relief was months away.

Pondering

How do you prepare yourself for medical procedures? How can a brief visit be such a blessing? Why is "brief" better sometimes than long visits?

Have you experienced a prickling thorn that God did not remove and you have to live with? How do you handle it with grace when He says, "My grace is sufficient"?

Chapter 12

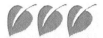

Phone Calls, the Sparrows, and a Fight

The salvation of the righteous comes from the Lord; He is their stronghold in time of trouble. Psalm 37:39

"Nothing sooner? We'll take it, but can you put us on a cancellation list?" Mayo Clinic had been at the top of all of our lists as the go-to place for the second opinion. But what now? I hung up feeling helpless; we had so little control of what, and when, and how. Would Wayne be destroyed by this cancer before we understood exactly what it was and the best way to fight it?

Monday the stent was inserted. Tuesday we met with Wayne's oncologist, Dr. C. He was kind, honest, and flexible; traits we came to treasure. He delivered the facts and a dose of hope.

"We have you scheduled for a brain scan on Friday, to see if it has spread there." He reviewed the aggressive nature of the cancer, warned us not to delay treatment, and offered some encouragement that it was treatable. Then he added, "A second opinion is fine, welcomed, but don't wait long."

Wednesday I made the call to Mayo and was told the first available appointment was three weeks away. *Too far away! Please God, help! What are we supposed to do?*

3 a.m. was becoming a regular wakeup time. I would sense Wayne getting out of bed and watch the digital numbers go to 3:01 . . . 3:02 . . . 3:03 . . . 3:16. Sometimes Wayne would sleep, but I could not seem to make it through the night. Finally, that week, after many early mornings of opening my eyes to sleep-robbing anxiety, I noticed a pattern. Most of

the time when I reluctantly looked at the glowing, green, digital numbers, I saw 3:16.

I still remember actually smiling when I finally got it: *For God so loved the world that He gave His one and only Son, that whoever believes in Him shall not perish, but have eternal life* (John 3:16). He loved us enough to die for us, had the power to rise and reign for us. He loved us enough for eternity. And He is loving us at this very moment. He is our stronghold.

Friday we went for the brain scan. I had been doing some reading and discovered the importance of having medical records available when a second opinion was scheduled. I asked for a copy of the scan.

"No problem, but you'll have to wait about 30 minutes." Wayne wanted out. All these appointments were grinding on him. The weight of this diagnosis combined with all the appointments was fraying his endurance. Reluctantly he sat down again in the waiting room.

"Please, just be patient. Just in case we need it." I hated insisting we wait, but I was holding out hope that somehow we would take it to Mayo with us. Minutes dragged by.

Finally, the technician came in with an envelope. "Here's the scan. It can be read on any computer." I slipped it into my purse and felt my eyes drawn to it over the weekend. It held secrets of health or disease, but what if I tried to read it when I knew I did not have the know-how? The scan seemed to taunt me.

Sunday afternoon the phone rang. Mostly I texted or emailed friends. Talking was exhausting. Tears were too ready to spill and often triggered by a compassionate voice. It took all my energy to hold them back. I saw the caller ID, a dear friend. I answered, "Hi."

"We want to offer you the company plane to go to Mayo Clinic. It's available Tuesday or Wednesday."

"Thanks, but the only appointment I could get is almost three weeks away. I don't know what we're going to do." I felt those pesky tears breaching the dam again.

"We're praying. Just let us know."

Monday morning I called Mayo again. They could move it up a week. But I had gotten a call that we had to meet with the radiologist on Friday.

Wayne had felt well enough to go to work for a few hours. I sat alone by the kitchen bar, my cell phone and the home phone on the counter next to my hand. *God, what's your number? Do you hear me?*

The cell phone rang. Jordan. I picked up. "Mom, did you try Mayo again?"

"Yes, but they can only move the appointment up a little and Dad has an appointment with the radiologist Friday. They want to begin radiation and chemo next week. Not looking good."

"Call them again . . . now."

"I just talked to them an hour ago."

"Trust me. I talked to a friend. Just call them."

"I'll pray about it and get back to you. Thanks for trying. Love you."

Lord, thank you for a son who cares so much about his dad. What do you want Father? This is too complicated for me. There are too many details, too many appointments, too much scheduling that has to coordinate. Help us! The home phone rang interrupting my prayer. Unable to ignore it, I checked caller ID and answered on the second ring.

"We just got a cancellation on Friday. Would your husband be able to be here at 7:30 in the morning?"

"Yes! We will! Thank You!" My voice was too loud.

She probably caught my desperation and quietly gave me the rest of the information we needed.

Months later Jordan shared a little of how God prompted him to make a call. *"They don't have any appointments available for a couple weeks. They will let us know if there are any cancellations."* Mom's voice was stressed, even for the last couple weeks.

Mom and Dad had been struggling with the decision of whether to start treatment locally, or get a second opinion at Mayo Clinic in Rochester, Minnesota. Everyone agreed that we wanted to start Dad's treatment as soon as possible. Every delay was another chance for the cancer to grow or spread. Nevertheless, despite the urgency to start treatment, the thought of a second set of eyes offered hope. Hope worth chasing down.

I could not read a PET scan and really didn't even know what radiation therapy was, but I knew I knew people who knew people. I made a phone call to a friend whose family had spent considerable time at Mayo. "Sure, Jordan. Shoot me your dad's specifics, and I'll see what I can do."

Friend's email to Mayo: 2:31 p.m., Sunday, February 1, 2015: "I'm contacting you to see if you might be able to help get my friend's father into Mayo to address his cancer issue. My friend is Jordan Bush and his father's name is Wayne William Bush. . . . I would very much appreciate any thing you might be able to do to get Wayne in as soon as possible. . . . I thank you for anything you might be able to do for Wayne and Jordan."

Hope.

Mayo's email to friend: 7:19 a.m., Monday, February 2, 2015: ". . . thank you very much for this note and I will be in contact with Jordan today."

After just a couple hours, I was excited and a bit nervous when my phone showed a 507 area code.

"Hi Jordan, this is __ with Mayo Clinic. Do you have a moment to chat?"

Yeah, I had a moment. I would have dropped everything and run to Rochester to have the conversation in person. While the incredibly kind and in-control woman on the other end of the line could not confirm anything due to Health Insurance Portability and Accountability Act (HIPAA) restrictions, she assured me that if her family was going through a health scare, Mayo was the place she would want them. She would follow up with a HIPAA release in the event, hypothetically of course, any of my family members became patients and wanted to authorize the release of information to me. I thanked her and immediately called Mom.

*****

"Give thanks with a grateful heart." Praise for the One who untangles knots and goes before us! The piano often beckons me to play my gratitude and the words of that song gave voice to the praises of my soul.

A few minutes later, I called Jordan back to share the news. Wayne's phone was in the truck while he worked. I texted the news, but plans had to be made before he even knew we were going.

I called the radiologist to change the Friday appointment. The secretary looked up Wayne's information and told me, "That appointment has already been changed to Monday. The doctor won't be here Friday. We were about to call you. Can you be here at 9:30 a.m. Monday?"

"We will."

Next call to the possibility of the plane. "No, I'm afraid it will be out of the state Friday, but let me make a call and get back to you."

Then to the Maps app to provide the directions and time needed; at best, an estimate depending on the snowy weather that could hit any of the five states we would be traveling in.

Text messages carried the news to the family with a request for prayers of thanksgiving and continued help covering all the details.

*****

Sparrows. As I paused after an hour, my mind turned to the sparrows. Fourteen years ago financial pressures bore down on our family, as they did on many families across the nation. My homebased business that had been doing well, dried up. An investment we thought was wise, ended up a complete loss. Expenses did not decline, but income did significantly. Turning back to teaching as a substitute brought in a little and planted a seed. Could I teach again after twenty-eight years out of the classroom?

6 a.m. calls requesting my presence in a variety of classrooms around the city led to experiences that confirmed God was leading me in this direction. One year later I began teaching at Calvin Christian High School during the day and an evening class on Monday nights for the University of Phoenix. My computer skills had to sharpen up quickly. Every evening was spent on lesson plans and grading. The alarm jarred me awake five mornings a week. I could get up, I could do the work, but I wondered if I could survive it.

One early morning in October I asked God, *How? How can I do all this? Are you with me?* Something flittered by my kitchen window as I sipped my first cup of caffeine for the day. A sparrow had found a safe nesting place near the window. As I watched, my mind began singing, *Why should I be discouraged? Why should the shadows fall? Why should my heart be lonely and long for heaven and home when Jesus is my portion? My constant friend is He: His eye is on the sparrow, and I know He watches me. His eye is on the sparrow, and I know He watches me.*

I had learned that old hymn as a child. It was one of my grandma's favorites. The author of that beloved hymn, Civilia D. Martin, a gifted writer, had died the year I was born. Oh, how her words blessed me that morning as she reminded me of God's faithfulness and care.

Of all the birds God created, why did He choose the plain, common sparrow to represent His goodness and compassion? Perhaps because they are so common. According to the Audubon Society, sparrows live around the globe, preferring to live near people. There are billions of them, and God says He knows each one (Luke 12:6).

From that moment on, sparrows became a symbol and a reminder that God did know me even though there are billions of people in the world. He knows us by name. He loves each one of us. My grandkids notice the sparrow figures scattered around our home, and know their message.

The morning of the Mayo call had been bright, a cold winter day capped with a blue sky. The sun shone through the arched window in our bathroom, casting a shadow of the top of the ornamental tree planted outside. That morning I had noticed the shadows of sparrows hopping across the branches. I had called Wayne in to look at the living wall art. Grace, a reminder that we often noticed in the months ahead.

*****

Wayne called on his lunch break in response to my text. We agreed to leave early Thursday morning to drive to Rochester. If the weather forecast predicted snow, we would allow two days and leave on Wednesday. But God was not finished revealing His detailed plan for this trip.

Tuesday morning felt like a transfusion for my body and spirit. I did something *normal*, I got a haircut. Kathy massaged my head in the shampoo bowl, trimmed my unruly locks, and blew them into order. I left there lifted and went to Bible Study.

I had written in my journal: *Life feels surreal—like everything is on hold. Cancer has invaded Wayne's body, our schedules, our thoughts, our energy, my goals, and even my dreams (fighting monsters and free falling out of disintegrating planes). What would happen to us without the prayers and love of family and friends? We are blessed, but at times I feel numb and focused only on this battle, waiting for time to pass—but the battle is just beginning.*

I needed my *storm sisters*, women who believe in the power of prayer and the reality of God's love. Women who seek to know Jesus and to live out the truth of His Word became instruments of God's grace to me. I met with a group of them at Calvary's Tuesday morning Bible study. My class with my leader Nancy Samra gave me the infusion of faith I needed that day, because life and its problems were waiting at the door. Turning my cell back on after class, I saw the message, "Call me" from Wayne.

"Are you okay?"

"Sure, but my car won't start, and it needs $1,100 in repairs."

Ouch! The lesson on Ephesians 6 about the armor of God came to mind. *Be strong in the Lord and in His mighty power* (Ephesians 6:10).

I'm glad you're okay, (*even though cancer is having a heyday in your body,* I thought but didn't say) and I'm glad they can fix the car."

After I said that, I remember feeling better. Yes, just speaking encouragement helped. Complaining seldom does and certainly doesn't change anything.

That afternoon while getting organized for our car trip to Mayo, my friend called. "We have a plane for you Friday morning!"

Early Friday morning we boarded the private jet with our two sons, who had again changed their schedules to be with us. I was struggling to keep hope rather than discouragement in my speech and on my heart. One of the pilots shared his story, "I had pancreatic cancer two years ago. Trust God, there is hope." Was it a coincidence that he was our pilot?

Pondering

Has God ever spoken to you in unexpected ways like the 3:16 clock numbers or the sparrows? Can you recall an event which seemed to fall into place when it was beyond your control? How do you feed your faith and encourage your heart?

Chapter 13

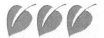

A Choice Must be Made

Trust in the Lord with all you heart and lean not on your own understanding; in all your ways acknowledge Him, and He will make your paths straight. Proverbs 3:5-6

As the plane sped down the runway in Grand Rapids, I fingered the dog tags hanging from the chain on my neck, a gift from Jordan to each member of the family. He would order many more as friends requested the symbol of solidarity growing around Wayne. They were engraved with the words: *God & Life are Good* on one tag and *Bush Strong* on the other. Long before it became the ubiquitous saying on hats and tee shirts, Wayne would answer, "Life is good," when asked, "How are you?" The kids had often teased him that he had started that trend.

Father, somehow make this journey, this cancer, count for the Kingdom. We know you are good. I will trust you. Prayers flitted through my thoughts as I gazed out of the window. The reality of the diagnosis and the need for this trip reminded me of the evil that showed up in our world in so many forms. How could—how would— God turn this to our good as He had promised us in Romans 8:28? *And we know that in all things God works for the good of those who love Him, who have been called according to His purposes.* I believed that and when I doubted, I would speak His promises aloud. Somehow He would use this experience for our family's good; and I prayed it would be for the good of His Kingdom.

The flight was short; soon we saw the ribbon of highway we would have traveled through the snow-covered fields of Minnesota. A taxi picked us up at the airport. "Text us this afternoon when you are ready to fly back. We'll meet you here." The pilots sent us off with a smile.

The taxi deposited us in front of the imposing Gonda Building standing tall in the center of Rochester. It is just one of the complex of buildings that make up the world famous Mayo Clinic. We joined a stream of people pouring into the enormous, marble lobby; people of different languages and cultural dress.

Soon we sat in a spacious waiting room on the ninth floor. Jordan and Justin were texting. They had promised the family frequent updates and included the light-hearted, like a picture of Jordan's fancy leather Italian dress shoes that Justin mocked.

Months later Justin shared his feelings about that trip: *Whether it was denial of how serious cancer is or an unnatural optimism, I was excited to go to Mayo. The thought that this cancer would give us a timeframe, would cut Dad's life short, never crossed my mind. Just knowing we were going to one of the best hospitals in the country reinforced my belief that Dad will fight this and win. I remember thinking God provided a jet, an opening at Mayo, and a doctor who has actually seen this type of cancer, how could all these pieces fall together only to get news no one would ever want to hear?*

"Wayne?" The attendant called his name and all four of us stood. She led us to a small exam room which we filled. The boys texted, "We're in, next text after this meeting."

Moments later the door opened to a short, compact figure dressed in a white, traditional, doctor's coat. He welcomed us as though we were guests coming to his home for dinner. He shook hands with the boys, chuckling up at their height. Then his eyes focused on Wayne.

"So, tell me what brought you here. How can we help you?" He had a file, but he waited for Wayne to answer. With gently probing questions he got to the heart of the matter. The three ring notebook I had assembled held the scans, reports, and analyses of the many tests which Wayne had undergone. I had a calendar sheet in the front with the date of each test. I simply added dates if Wayne hesitated and handed over the latest scan we had waited for the previous Friday.

This was the beginning of our relationship with Dr. B, a man we came to trust and look to as one of God's answers to our many prayers. He gave each of his patients the gift of his time, focus, and brilliant mind. I noticed that during our many visits he would search Wayne's face and ask if he had any questions about the medical information and choices that had to be made. His explanations were thorough, including a review of the PET scans, latest lab results, and when decisions about treatment had to be made he shared on-line studies he had researched. He concluded many of our visits with: "You are in charge, Wayne. I'll follow your wishes." He empowered his patients with information and respect.

After the initial questions, he examined Wayne and noticed a cyst the other doctors had dismissed. "I would like a friend of mine, a dermatologist, to look at that. He's up on the twelfth floor. Is that okay?"

Dr. D, another gifted doctor, examined Wayne. "I would like to excise that and have a biopsy. That may be the root of your cancer. I can do that right now as soon as the paper work is completed by the business office."

All eyes turned to Wayne for his decision. I forced myself to wait, though I wanted to insist, *Do it!* One of the answers to my prayers for God's guidance was a little more self-control. I needed to be still and wait; something my natural impulses did not desire. Later on I learned how wise that resolution was because it is essential for the patient to be as actively involved in decision making as possible.[1]

"If you think it's important, I'll do it." The boys and I sighed with relief.

Justin stood in line with me as I waited my turn at the business counter. It was only a few minutes, but seemed longer. "Can I help you?"

I explained the situation and gave her our insurance cards. "We'll contact them, but meanwhile you'll have to put down __ (for us, a substantial amount of money).

Insurance. A fact of life that controls a lot of decisions and expenses. I had gotten permission from our insurance company for this visit which was out-of-network, but not for any treatments or procedures. I had transferred money from our savings account before we left in case of added expenses. There would be just enough. I reached for my check book as she turned to a coworker adding, "The rules and regulations are complex."

A moment later she returned, "I was wrong. We only need $100 because you have a Medicare card. I'll let the doctor know, and you take this with you."

Thankful, we rushed back upstairs with the necessary papers.

Wayne was already prepped and lying on the surgical bed when the nurse led me to him. A kiss, a quick hug, a whispered, "I love you. Be good and don't say anything too crazy," and I was shown to the waiting room where the boys were already sitting.

Time passed, and we waited. I had brought some food for the boys, but found I couldn't eat. Ironically, it was the boys who reminded me to drink something at least. Again tables turned.

Several hours later we were back in Dr. B's office. He came in with a team of doctors and introduced us to a radiologist and a surgeon. "At Mayo, we often work in teams and everyone gives their insights. I have already talked with Dr. D upstairs and understand the recommendations he made to you. These doctors have looked at your information, and I'll present you with your options for treatment and answer any questions. Wayne, you'll make the decision how you want us to proceed."

"We think your cancer is Merkel cell carcinoma which is a rare aggressive cancer. It is a subdivision of the small cell diagnosis you received. The biopsy will verify that. I'll call you Monday with the lab results." He then went on to present the three very different protocols that had been recommended, including the options we had been given in Grand Rapids. It amazed me how patient and thorough he was in explaining complex medical issues to four nonmedical people.

"So Wayne, how do you want to proceed?"

It was like standing in front of three doors. One of them held the best option for Wayne. Which one? Once we walked through that door . . .

Earlier I had heard Dr. D's recommendation; I knew the Grand Rapids plan, and Dr. B felt strongly about a third protocol. While I had waited to see Wayne after his procedure upstairs my mind had twisted with fear. In anguish tears filled a tissue as I pleaded with God for *His* plan and for unity of minds among the family members and the doctors. The boys and I had prayed together, "God make our path straight and bring us to unity. Reveal your will to each of us."

Silence weighed down on us as we waited for Wayne's decision. When he firmly committed to Dr. B's recommendation, I saw Jordan and Justin relax with relief and nod their heads in agreement. Later, we shared the moment we each felt convicted that one approach was the best; that was the moment we waited for Wayne's answer. God had answered our prayer for unity of mind. Now what about the doctors in Grand Rapids? We would find out Monday when we met with the radiologist.

Justin recalls, *Towards the end of the day when we heard Dr. B's plan on how to fight this, I was reassured even more that cancer will not beat Dad and won't break our family apart. Whether Dad was masking how he really felt inside, I don't know; I remember he was always positive and even would crack jokes with the hospital staff. His attitude helped me stay in a better place that day.*

Dr. B promised to send a full report to our oncologist in Grand Rapids and give him a call. As we rose to leave, I wanted to hug him for his kindness, patience, and encouragement. Somehow I knew he preferred a sincere handshake and thank you.

The boys texted the pilots that we would be at the airport soon. They were waiting, and we shared our experiences before boarding. After I gave them our small thank you gifts, the pilot who had recovered from pancreatic cancer took a moment to tell me a little about his journey and what he had done. He encouraged me to call his wife and gave me her number. "There are things you can do to help Wayne. Talk to my wife. She did a lot of research. It made a difference."

Pondering

How can something like the dog tags help strengthen a family? What other ideas are there? How do you and your family make decisions? Do your medical caregivers give you sufficient information and respect to make wise choices?

Proverbs 3:5-6 is an excellent verse to memorize for any decision. Do you have other verses that strengthen you in that process?

[1]Turner, Ph.D., Kelly A. Radical Remission: Surviving Cancer Against All Odds. New York: HarperCollins, 2014.

Chapter 14

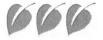

The What Else of Eating, Seeking, Learning, Drawing Closer

I will lead the blind by ways they have not known, along unfamiliar paths I will guide them; I will turn the darkness into light before them and make the rough places smooth. These are the things I will do; I will not forsake them. Isaiah 42:16

At 5:00 p.m. we pulled into our driveway. Had all this been accomplished in one day? We had a clearer picture of the enemy having seen the scans and heard the reports. The news was grim, but God . . . God was with us.

The pilot's conversation with me reinforced an idea I had that there was more that we could do. The human body designed by the Creator has a powerful tool: the immune system which fights off disease. How could we strengthen Wayne's immune system to squelch the cancer cells and deal with the side effects of the chemo therapies and radiation? What additional edge could we employ? Those questions had provoked prayers for wisdom, searches on the internet, and the purchase of various books. While I was searching, Stephanie, Meredith, and Leah were also diving into their resources hunting for information.

Saturday arrived and the family gathered again. Stephanie and Paul had packed the kids and their yellow lab, Max, for the two hour trip through the snow. The backyard turned into a winter wonderland as they made snowmen, forts, and snow angels. The back hall filled with snowsuits, boots, scarves and mittens.

For supper the grandkids and I rolled out bread dough, their aprons and hands becoming dusty with flour. They piled on the meats, cheeses, and spices, and folded them up to make Stromboli. We bumped hips as everyone helped make salads, set the table, get more chairs. It was crowded, noisy, and the aroma of baking bread and spices filled the air. I paused, leaned against the counter, and watched to savor this good moment, this gift that filled my senses and fed my soul.

After supper while the grandgirls went downstairs to play and the hockey game entertained the boys, Stephanie, Meredith, Leah, and I had a few minutes to share some of our research.

A few weeks earlier I had attended one of the events at Calvin College's January Series. The one day Wayne did not have appointments and I could attend, the speaker happened to be Dr. David Katz, author of *Disease Proof: Slash Your Risk of Heart Disease, Cancer, and Diabetes, and More—by 80 Percent*. Was that a coincidence? I bought his book. I also found *Anticancer: A New Way of Life* by Dr. David Servan-Schreiber, MD, PhD. (For a list of resources we used and continue to use, see the Resource page in the back of the book.)

Stephanie's research confirmed the benefits of an adjusted diet strong on certain fruits and vegetables. She had recipes for me. Meredith had discovered the benefits of essential oils, especially frankincense, and had brought her diffuser and the oil with her. Leah, a personal trainer, shared her knowledge of the importance of exercise. Her comments reinforced our trips to Rivertown Mall to join the mall walkers and stroll two miles in the climate-controlled setting, much appreciated in the wintery months in Michigan. All of us knew that adding to our arsenal of defensive, immune-building tactics could make a difference.

Their enthusiasm reinforced my efforts. Over the months ahead I continued to research and learn more ways to minimize the effects of the treatments and maximize Wayne's strength. Some things were simple, like keeping Nikken magsteps (patented magnetic insoles, see the Resource page) in Wayne's shoes; for him, this seemed to prevent any neuropathy, a common side effect of the powerful chemotherapies he received. He also benefitted from other products like their comforter which helped reduce his nausea.

I was open to ideas, listened to suggestions, prayed about them, and implemented them if Wayne was willing. I admit that sometimes my efforts were less than appreciated. One night several weeks into treatment, Wayne came home after being able to work that day. I had a new recipe of vegetables cooking. He walked in, gave me a hug, sniffed, and stepped back into the garage. "Please get rid of that. I can't stand the smell; I'm gagging."

Disappointed, but accepting that chemo had changed his taste buds and tolerance, I dumped that meal in the garbage disposal. I learned to balance between super healthy and edible. The bottom line is that we modified the way we ate and explored new foods and healthier options. My library of resources grew.

Besides the physical components, we learned about the emotional and spiritual factors that play significant roles in the day to day journey of dealing with cancer. One of Wayne's doctors had been blunt: "Wayne, we're going to do all we can for you, but if there is anything you need to get in order, you should do that. If there's anything you had hoped to do, do it."

The proverbial bucket list came to mind. That was the lighthearted way of looking at it. The bottom line is that we were confronted with the fragile nature of life and the possibility of death happening sooner than we had anticipated. That is the soul-searching, gut-wrenching level.

Life *is* good, because God is good. He breathed into us the breath of life and by our very nature we are designed to desire life and the complex longing for relationship—with God and with people. Cancer is destructive and isolating. It wasn't that long ago that doctors hid the truth from their patients, and patients, if they knew, hid the truth from their families and friends. Perhaps they considered that a kindness and a way to focus on life rather than death. Thankfully today more truth is revealed. I was determined to face the truth no matter how hard it was and do whatever I could to encourage life. I think I was influenced by events in my grandparents' lives.

My mother's parents had a long, loving marriage. They were only 20 years old when they married in the Netherlands and decided to carry their hopes and dreams a world away to the United States. Grandpa planned to put his new bride on the best ship available even though they would have to travel second class. His plans were changed when his mother pleaded with him: "You are going so far away, and I may never see you again. My last request to you is to sail on a good Dutch ship."

Out of respect, he listened. He turned in his tickets and bought new ones. They arrived in New York City in the spring of 1912 on the Holland American Line. Their original tickets had been for the newest British ship, the *Titanic*.

They settled near the harbor where they landed in Hoboken, New Jersey. Maybe that start to their married life is part of what made their faith and love so strong.

I remember I was in high school when Grandma got sick. She suffered from colon cancer which racked her body with pain. Grandpa would sit by her and hold her hand. When she died my mom told me he asked the doctor, "Why didn't you tell me she had cancer? You just said it was tumors. I thought she would get better." His grief was deep.

Facing the possibility of Wayne's death felt like facing my own. Our lives are deeply entwined and the peace we feel in each other's presence has been forged on the trials we have faced together. Over the years we have developed routines of sharing responsibilities and making space for each other's needs. The simple tasks of daily life are easier because there is a spirit of mutual kindness. Days have more joy because we share them. How would I ever sleep through the night if I couldn't feel the warmth of his body close to mine?

Even as I searched for ways to help him physically, I also sought for ways to help us both emotionally. I knew that a positive attitude is one of the most essential tools in helping our immune systems. Science has proven the detrimental impact of prolonged stress and anxiety on the body and the benefits of a positive attitude. But even before I had read that, I remembered what God said about worry: "Don't!" and what He said about fear: "Don't" There are over 330 references in the Bible about this. Clearly, God recognizes the problem we have and gave us many verses to claim when we struggle. And it is a struggle.

One of my favorites that kept playing through my mind was Philippians 4:4-7. *Rejoice in the Lord always. I will say it again: Rejoice! Let your gentleness be evident to all. The Lord is near. Do not be anxious about anything, but in every situation, by prayer and petition, with thanksgiving, present your requests to God. And the peace of God, which transcends all understanding, will guard your hearts and your minds in Christ Jesus.*

We had to deliberately choose how we were going to live each day. We had to be thankful on purpose. The benefit of choosing to rejoice and choosing to be thankful would be peace. Easier said than done; it was a daily, hourly, sometimes minute by minute decision. I learned quickly that not only what we fed our stomachs mattered. We had to feed our souls to nourish our emotions.

We started with our Bibles, and then God gave us witnesses who had experienced the peace we needed. They shared their stories which watered the fragile hope and peace that had been assaulted by fear. The first morning I had returned to Tuesday morning Bible study after Wayne's diagnosis, I met Susan Sorensen. She leads the women's ministry at our church. Our meeting was an interesting coincidence—*coincidence* defined as God-directed.

Something in her compassionate nature led me to share our need for prayer. She asked me to come to her office after class. That's when I learned she too had wrestled with cancer which had attacked her body

68

twice. Those experiences resulted in the book she handed me: *Praying Through Cancer: Set Your Heart Free from Fear* part of which she had written and edited.

This book blessed my thoughts and watered my parched spirit with hope. It is a collection of 90 devotions written by women who have and are dealing with a soul-wrenching fight with cancer.

The first one was written by Kay Warren, Rick Warren's wife. (He is the senior pastor of Saddleback Church and author of *The Purpose Driven Life*.) Her prayer lingered with me long after I read it: *God, how can I ever thank You for showing up when I need You the most? I am never alone! You promise to be my refuge and my strength, my ever present help in trouble. . . . You will fulfill Your purpose for me. . . . May this furnace of testing show the true colors of my faith in You, and may I come forth as gold.*[2]

I looked up every Bible reference she gave for the promises proclaimed in that prayer, underlined them in my Bible, and claimed those promises as ours. Each devotional in that book, many written by Susan, subdued fear and fed faith.

Wayne found solace in Sarah Young's *Jesus Calling*. In the introduction, she explains how this devotional book is a product of her own deep needs and time with God. She also shares the Bible verses and devotionals that spoke to her heart and prompted her to write from the perspective of Jesus. The January 22 entry seemed to be written directly to us: *Strive to trust me in more and more areas of your life. Anything that tends to make you anxious is a growth opportunity. . . . Don't waste energy regretting the way things are or thinking about what might have been. Start at the present moment—accepting things exactly as they are—and search for My way in the midst of those circumstances.*[3]

Words, the power of words to comfort, instruct, guide. Words delivered to us in conversations and sermons; words delivered in books, and text messages, and cards; words floating on the melodies of songs. We prayed for discernment to clearly trust the words God was providing.

They revealed a way for us to actively participate in God's will for Wayne's life, and if He chose, in his death.

When confronted with questions about life and death, the underlying questions really become: "What matters? What helps?" If they can be answered, then we know how to live each day we are given. As I wrestled with thoughts of Wayne's death, at first the pain felt unbearable, and the tears welled up often. Gradually God wove His promises and comfort through my troubled spirit.

Life in all of its joy and complexity, that's what mattered to me. God reminded me it mattered to Him as well. So much that He had given His

Son so I could go beyond my finite understanding of life and experience eternal life (John 3:16).

In His prayer the night before He was crucified, Jesus defined the eternal life He was offering to us. *Now this is eternal life: that they know you, the only true God, and Jesus Christ, whom you have sent* (John 17:3). We prayed with Paul *that the God of our Lord Jesus Christ, the glorious Father, would give us the Spirit of wisdom and revelation, so that we could know Him better* (Ephesians 1:17). *Jesus said, "I am the resurrection and the life. The one who believes in me will live, even though they die, and whoever lives by believing in me will never die* (John 11:25-26).

We believe in Jesus so we needed to understand how He would fulfill the other important promise He made about eternal life starting as soon as we believe. Cancer attacked our joy. Jesus understands that. He called evil like this a thief. *The thief comes only in order to steal and kill and destroy. I came that they may have and enjoy life, and have it in abundance (to the full, till it overflows)* (John 10:10 Amplified Bible).

What helped us reclaim joy each day was the presence of God, the faith, hope, and love which He gave us. He reminded me of the catechism question and answer I had learned as a child: *What is your only comfort in life and in death? That I am not my own but belong— body and soul, in life and in death—to my faithful Savior Jesus Christ. . . . Therefore, by His Holy Spirit He also assures me of eternal life, and makes me heartily willing and ready from now on to live for Him.*[4]

He gave us more sensitive spirits to see how He was providing for us on our journey. *Even though we were walking through the shadow of death, we did not need to live in the fear of evil. For the Lord, our Shepherd, was with us. His rod and His staff they comforted us. He prepared a table before us in the presence of our enemy. Surely goodness and mercy followed us all the days of our lives and we will dwell in the house of the Lord forever* (Psalm 23).

We had to discover what was the *goodness and mercy* God had in store for us each day. We always found our best peace in time with God, followed by the relationships we had with our family and friends. Time together and communication brought encouragement.

As we gave thanks for each good gift of each good moment, He opened our eyes to His care, restored our souls, gave us peace, and delivered joy. Our love and appreciation for our children and grandchildren showered us with delight. Old hymns like "What a Friend We Have in Jesus" and newer songs like "10,000 Reasons" and "Blessed be the Name" by Matt Redman lifted our spirits and echoed in our minds. We discovered that being grateful fostered more hope than grumbling.

Reaching out to someone else in need delivered more grace. A game of Sequence was a great worry distractor.

He taught us to breathe in His grace and breathe out our praise. Even on the toughest days, He wrapped us close in the blanket of His love. He is faithful.

Pondering

Where do you go for answers when you are confronted with health problems? Aside from the medicine you are given, how do you participate in your own healing? How do you sort through the advice you find?

What do you do to nourish your emotions and your soul? What matters to you? What brings you comfort?

[2] Sorensen, Susan, and Laura Geist. Praying Through Cancer: Set Your Heart Free from Fear. Nashville, Thomas Nelson, 2006, 2.

[3] Young, Sarah. Jesus Calling. Nashville, TN: Thomas Nelson, 2004, 23.

[4] Heidelberg Catechism/Christian Reformed Church. Google, https://www.crcna.org/welcome/beliefs/confessions/heidelberg-catechism. Lord's Day 1, Q&A 1.

Three Generations Fight Cancer Together

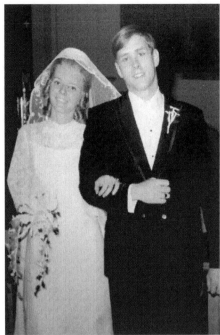

Our wedding day in New Jersey, December 26, 1969

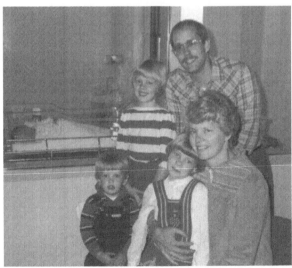

First family picture with all four kids, Grand Rapids, Michigan

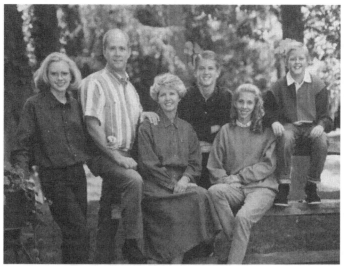

The family growing up
(Photo by Harley Photography. Used by Permission)

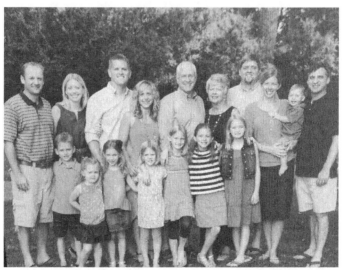

Growing Family: This picture taken in Grandville, Michigan just
a few months before the diagnosis
(Photo by Laura Hoeksema. Used by Permission)

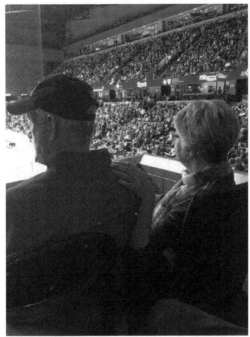

Griffins' hockey game at Van Andel Arena in
Grand Rapids three days after getting the news

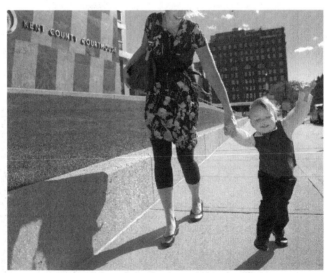

Meredith and Andrew on Adoption Day,
Kent County Courthouse, Grand Rapids

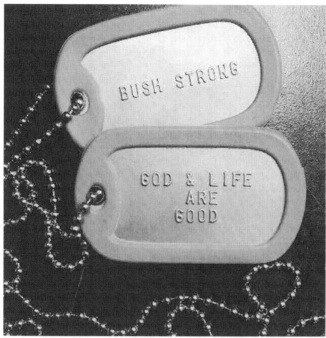

Dog tags Jordan ordered for family and friends

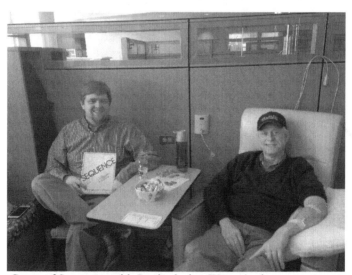

Game of Sequence with Justin during Wayne's chemo treatment
at Lemmen-Holton in Grand Rapids

Three Generations Fight Cancer Together

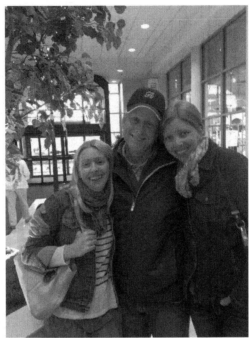

Stephanie and Meredith with us at Mayo Clinic, Rochester, Minnesota

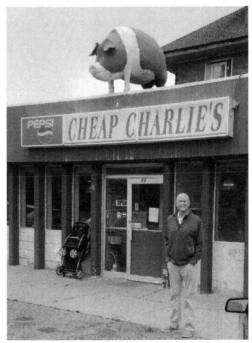

Father's Day at a local spot in Rochester

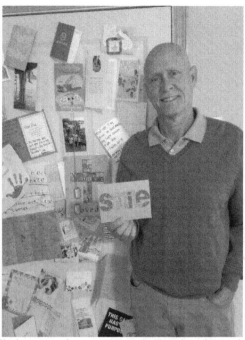

Family love taped on our Hope Lodge door in Rochester

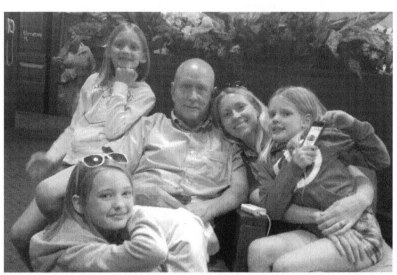

Stephanie and the girls waiting with us for three hours until the radiation beeper finally flashed at Mayo Clinic

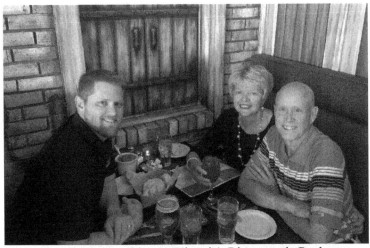

Jordan celebrating with us at Victoria's Ristorante in Rochester

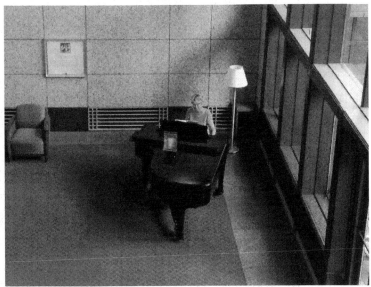

Elaine playing one of Mayo's grand pianos

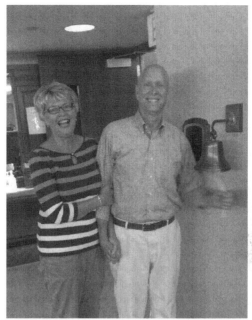

Ringing the bell to celebrate the final radiation treatment at Mayo Clinic

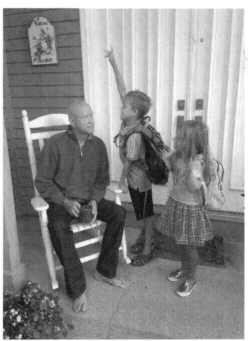

Early morning on the front porch in Grandville, the first day of school

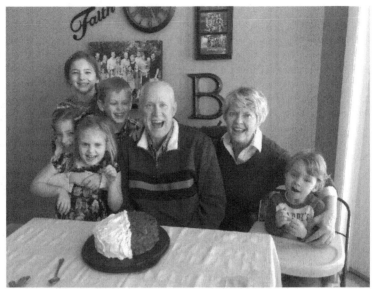

Half-way-there celebration cake in the fall during treatment in Grand Rapids

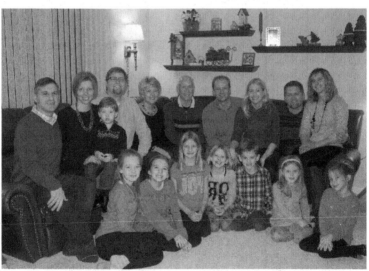

Family Christmas Celebration in Grandville, December 26, 2015

Chapter 15

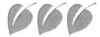

Treatment, Stress Fractures, and a Beam of Hope

You, Lord, keep my lamp burning; my God turns my darkness into light. With your help I can advance against a troop; with my God I can scale a wall. . . . It is God who arms me with strength and keeps my way secure. Psalm 18:28-29, 32

One more hurdle to face Monday morning before treatment began. Dr. M introduced himself, sat on a swivel stool facing Wayne, and after a few questions addressed the issue that concerned us, "I think we should wait with the radiation until we see the results of the chemo treatment. I've seen the Mayo report." Relief and gratitude. Everyone agreed.

Tuesday morning I packed snacks, a Sudoku book, a novel, and a game as well as the green notebook and 3-ring binder. We had been warned that it would be a long day. Car after car pulled up to the entrance of Lemmen-Holton Cancer Pavilion. Warmly-dressed parking attendants whisked cars away, allowing patients a short walk to the door. We would come to appreciate that kindness through the long Michigan winter.

This visit, the powerful chemotherapy drugs would begin to drip into Wayne's veins. Everything in me wanted to run. We had been prepped with a long list of side effects that could happen. The word *poison* came to mind. We sat in the large waiting room, and I studied the impact cancer and its treatments were having on our fellow pilgrims. There were wheelchairs and walkers for legs too weak to support themselves. There were bodies gaunt in appearance.

We had been warned that Wayne's taste buds would change, that nausea was common, that "every calorie you can get down and keep down is a good calorie." No wonder people referred to cancer as a war! It took incredible courage to fight this enemy day after day. It assaulted the body, the mind, and the spirit. It assaulted the family.

So why were all these people here? The bottom line is life is precious and worth fighting for. Cancer could be attacked, and there were people who were willing to help us. There were smiles in that waiting room. There was hope. Perhaps what I noticed the most was the patient endurance. As I wrestled with my anxieties, I reminded myself to choose my attitude. If I was going to be of any help to Wayne, I had to refocus my thoughts. This was the mental skirmish I was fighting.

Wayne was better at this than I was. When his name was called, he got up, smiled at the attendant, and started chatting with her as I trailed behind. We entered a large room with open cubicles. Each one held a comfortable recliner, a chair, a small television, a tray, and the object that gave me a chill—the IV pole to hold the bag of chemo.

His veins are strong so Wayne had chosen to avoid a port in his chest. Although the vein was clearly bulging the nurse had trouble getting a line started. After several pokes with the needle, my teeth were clenched, but Wayne remarked, "I'm going to have to change my first impression that you're a really good nurse." They both laughed. I didn't.

Finally, the needle was in place and taped to his arm. "It will stay in place for the week. We'll bandage it well before you go home today." I was relieved he would not have to go through this the next day, but uncomfortable with the thought of this intruder poking out of his arm. What if I bumped it?

Sitting there is both so personal and so communal. Each cubicle held warriors. Some were alone; some with a family member or friend. Some read; the books often settled on their laps as they dozed. Chemo is exhausting. Some played games or chatted with a spouse or friend who had come. Only a few turned to the television for distraction. Some, like me, just sat quietly.

Perhaps people get used to it; I never did. I was never able to focus on reading or writing or even talking much. Often Wayne and I sat together there in quietness, simply reaching for the other's hand once in a while. Sometimes he would reach for my hand and say, "I'm glad you're here. I need you." Other times it was simply, "I love you."

I could not imagine being anywhere else. Friends would offer to go and sit with Wayne as the weeks passed, but I couldn't accept their offers. Months later I agreed to his twin brother Warren going with Wayne while I stayed home. It surprised me how hard it was.

So it began. Hours of waiting while assault troops were deployed into Wayne's bloodstream to destroy the cancer cells. I watched as the IV bag drained and heard Wayne assure the nurses who checked with him that he was fine.

One hour into the treatment a familiar face came around the corner. Jordan worked downtown and came over to sit with us for a couple of hours. I knew he was busy, but it was easy to let him stay and distract us. He took a picture on his cell phone and texted it out to the family. That became a regular habit of each of his siblings as they took turns coming down to Lemmen-Holton.

Justin shared, *I thought I'd have more of an emotional reaction seeing Dad hooked up and knowing what was going through his body, but since we were sending out pictures every time someone went to hang out with Dad, I just felt happy to be there. I felt good being able to play Sequence and being a distraction from why we were there.*

One morning before chemo I had to run to Meijer, the local grocery store. Hurrying to the self-checkout lane, I noticed a bucket of carnations. That reminded me of an idea from the book *Fight Back with Joy*. I grabbed a dozen of them. Wayne was waiting to go when I got home. "Just a minute, I need some ribbon and a scissors."

While the chemo bag emptied, I tied a ribbon around each carnation and delivered them to fellow warriors. I admit I thought it was a little silly when I began. By the time I returned to Wayne, I had tears in my eyes. That small gesture had brought smiles, tears, and expressions of gratitude that humbled me. One lady sitting by herself grinned and said, "My first flower on the last day of chemo! What a blessing!" Oh, what a lesson I learned that day!

Four long days of heavy chemo and then a Neulasta shot. The shot was supposed to help his bone marrow, but with the help there also came a long list of potential problems. The benefits seemed to outweigh the risks. Another choice we had to make. Round 1 completed.

For two weeks Wayne would not have any more chemo. For two weeks we would wait for another scan. For two and a half weeks we would wait for the results of Round 1. For two and a half weeks we tried to ignore the elephant in the room and just be normal. Waiting doesn't come easy. Anxiety creeps in the cracks, especially during the night. Defenses seem to be lower then.

The stent would wake Wayne up several times a night. Quietly he slipped out of bed, but I almost always woke up. When he knew his mind would not let him rest, he would push a pillow against my back. He knew I would miss his closeness and hoped to cover his absence. It didn't work very often.

I would pray, quote verses to myself, sing in my head, and finally get up to see how he was doing. Often he was reading *Jesus Calling* by Sarah Young or Ed Dobson's book, *Prayers and Promises When Facing a Life-Threatening Illness*. Our former pastor kept ministering to us through the words he had written during his journey with ALS. After an hour, some peace restored, Wayne returned to bed and sleep.

At first there seemed to be few side effects from the chemo, then I noticed his appetite was changing. I watched him at supper as he took a small bite, put his fork down, chewed, and hesitated before picking up the fork again. Food was losing its appeal.

The scan was scheduled at Spectrum's West Pavilion just a few minutes from our home. We were told we would get the results the following week. I asked for a copy of the scan. Again I knew better than to try to read it. As soon as we were home I wrote a note to Dr. B at Mayo Clinic, tucked the note and scan in an envelope, and headed through the falling snow to the post office. It was the end of February. We had been in this war for two months. How many more would there be?

*****

Our favorite day of the week was Sunday for several reasons. One of them was Jim Samra, our pastor at Calvary. He was preaching a series on Hebrews. We learned that the book was a story of Jesus' journey and how that journey paralleled ours. He showed us how the book started at the end of the story with Christ's victory before unfolding the painful journey of Jesus' life here on earth. It concluded with the giants of the faith who had endured terrible trials.

He challenged us to be people of faith and remember that God knows our suffering and our victory is sure no matter the circumstances. His words were like transfusions for our spirits, strengthening us for the week ahead.

One Sunday morning Wayne and I walked to the front after the service to thank him for ministering to us. He placed his hand on Wayne's shoulder and prayed over him. A gift of grace.

The aroma of roasting meat greeted us when we got home. Sunday dinners served after the morning service have a long tradition in our families going back several generations. Our children and grandchildren enjoy them too and often join us for meals including items like mashed potatoes and gravy, green salads, and red Jello salads packed with strawberries and mandarin oranges, vegetables, homemade pumpkin bread, and desserts of root beer floats or vanilla fudge ice cream cones for the kids, and apple pie for the adults.

William has a thing for his Papa and loved coming over to our house on Sunday. From the time he was two years old he would greet me when I answered the door with, "Where's Papa?" One Sunday his family got to our house before we did so I sent Wayne in first. Papa got his big hug and kiss. I was waiting to hear, "Where's Grandma?" Instead, when he spotted me coming in he pointed to Wayne and announced, "Here's Papa!"

Another Sunday when he was three years old I discovered that he loved Jello salads loaded with fruit. So, of course, Jello salads became a fairly regular menu item on Sunday. He was four when he asked me as soon as he arrived, "Grandma, did you bake a Jello for today?"

"Check the refrigerator." I smiled and watched his discovery. When he saw the familiar green Tupperware he took it out and hugged it. Before I could stop him he ran into the family room with its light carpeting that had just been cleaned to show his prize to Papa. Thankfully the lid held tight.

At his next sleep-over visit, we made Jello together, and he learned there was no baking involved, just lots of stirring which he loved to do,

William's mom Leah shared: *I did not feel like I was needed on the "front lines" so to speak. There seemed to be enough immediate family and friends who wanted to sit with Dad during his treatments and be present at those times. I felt called to continue praying and supporting Jordan as he was closer to the action.*

I also made sure to keep my kids informed on Papa's changing appearance which honestly did not seem to affect them or me much at all.

Some of the best memories I have during this terrible treatment season were our Sunday Sequence games. It felt so good to spend many weekends together and allow ourselves to laugh! I remember the day it became comfortable to start jokingly using the term "playing the cancer card." We all laughed so hard trying to think of the things we could score for Dad since his body was the one going through cancer. The conversation culminated in somewhat spontaneously booking a trip to Boyne Mountain for a family vacation in the summer!

Those Sundays were such an encouragement to me and our family and our laughter brought so much hope during that hard time. It was especially heart-warming to see you and Dad allowing yourselves some joy in the midst of your pain.

Thursday, February 26 Wayne's veins again accepted the IV. This time the solution would reveal the growth or regression of the cancer in his body. I had registered his online patient portal where results would be posted. Every day I checked—nothing. I tried Lemmen-Holton; nothing yet. The report would also be sent to his primary care physician. On Monday I called his office. He was gone for the day. The doctor on call was my doctor. I explained what I was looking for and the receptionist said she would pass on my request.

Hours passed. Each ring of the phone that day raised my heart rate. Late afternoon it rang again. "Hi, this is Dr. I's office. We have the results you asked about. Do you want me to read it to you?"

"Please."

First a description of the procedure and the medication used during the scan, followed by medical jargon I didn't understand. Then a note no cancer was found in the lungs. More medical terms.

"Stop! Please read that last sentence again." One word I was listening for—*regression.*

"Would you please tell me if that term has any other meaning in the medical world than what it means to me? Is this good news?"

"Your doctor will explain everything. But, yes, this is good news."

A glimmer of hope!

Pondering

What helps you pass time during periods of waiting? How can food be a comfort? How can you make room for laughter? Do you have games almost all ages can play? We often turned to Sequence and Dominoes.

Chapter 16

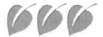

Another Season, Another Treatment Plan, Another Act of Obedience

Even to your old age and gray hairs I am He, I am He who will sustain you. I have made you and I will carry you; I will sustain you and I will rescue you. Isaiah 46:4

Patches of melting snow marked the end of winter. Wayne finished his third heavy round of chemo still smiling, but thinner and completely bald. The second scan revealing the chemo's impact on the cancer was scheduled for the day before Good Friday. No results until the following week.

"Is it okay if we come for Easter? I know Dad's tired." Stephanie had noticed, probably more than the rest of us who saw him every day, or at least weekly, that her Dad's physical appearance and his stamina were declining. She had packed up her family every other weekend since January and would see what two more weeks of the fight cost him.

"Honey, you are a dose of joy for both of us! Please come," I urged her.

One of Wayne's doctors had told us we might see the greatest response after the first round and subsequent rounds could be less effective. The first scan had revealed a great response, but now Wayne's body was weaker. Would this new scan still show regression? It would be a long weekend waiting for results and then what? More chemo? Radiation? Surgery?

Michigan winters reluctantly yield to the warmth of spring, but Easter morning arrived with blue skies and find-your-spring-coat temperatures.

We had missed several Sunday services due to heavy colds and bad weather, so walking into church that morning held a special sweetness of coming home. As our pastor greeted the congregation with "He is risen," we responded with renewed conviction, "He is risen indeed."

As in January the family met us at church to worship together. My friend Debbie joined us as well. We love her like a family member and had grieved deeply with her when her husband had suddenly died. She looked at me with tears in her eyes as we sang, "Christ the Lord is risen today." I reached for her hand. There was a tightness in my chest of gratitude—an overflowing of praise for God's faithfulness through the painful seasons of our lives, a deeper awareness of His presence in the brokenness, disappointments, and struggles. We carried scars, wounds, and the paper cuts of daily living, but because He lives, we can live and breathe today. We can experience joy.

After Sunday dinner joy arrived at the sight of eight grandchildren poised on the front porch, waiting for the countdown to find the 150 eggs their Papa, dads, and uncles had placed in the front, side, and back yards. Grace, Lauren, and Aubrey, the oldest grandchildren, had told the younger ones to pick up the easy-to-spot eggs. "We'll find the hard ones!"

The sun had warmed the afternoon to jacketless temperatures that infused us all with spring fever. Two year old Andrew ran at the start with his cousins and picked up the first bright blue egg he spotted. He shook it and promptly sat down on the grass to investigate what was hidden inside. Finding a few M & M's, which he devoured, spurred him on to find more eggs. Within minutes all but one egg was found.

Uncle Justin insisted there was one more remaining. After some pleading he agreed to "You're getting hotter. You're getting colder," to guide them to the hard-to-spot egg.

Then the counting, opening, and trading of stickers, candy, and small toys began.

Worship, laughter, and love did their best to build us up for what lay ahead that week.

*****

"Hi, how are you feeling today?" Dr. C. began Wayne's Thursday appointment.

"Good."

Wayne's answer, I knew, really depended on the report resting on the doctor's lap.

"Your scan shows further regression." Pause.

Relief, but a sense that there was more. I held my breath.

"Not as much as the first time. We'll continue with another round of chemo."

Wayne was quiet as we waited in the lobby for our car.

"It is good news." I tried to reassure both of us. "You are moving in the right direction."

The following Tuesday evening Dr. B. from Mayo called. "I went over the report. The surgeon and I believe you should return to Mayo in May for tests and possibly surgery. You are making progress, but this cancer is serious."

Wednesday Wayne had his usual blood draw. When his name was called to begin the next round of chemo his favorite nurse's hands were empty. She did not have the chemo. "Sorry, we'll have to wait until next week. Your counts are too low to begin."

"What can he do to build them up?"

"Rest and wait."

We waited again for our car in the lobby. The chill of winter had returned. Neither of us said much. I leaned against his side.

*****

Only four months had passed since we began this journey. It felt much longer. Our lives seemed to be on hold. Friends talked about summer plans, vacations, trips, work. There was a time when I enjoyed making plans, dreaming about the future, planning projects. Now my emotions felt crushed under the weight of cancer and all its demands. Some days I caught myself simply sitting, staring, unable to do anything.

For my sake and for Wayne's I learned the important lesson of reaching out beyond the family to a greater circle of support. We had joined a small group at church in the fall. We met a couple times a month on Sunday night: some food, fellowship, study time, and prayer. At first we were strangers, then pleasant acquaintances, then friends, and then storm troopers for each other raising the sacrifice of prayer for the needs we shared. I learned that a quick text to the group would be followed by greater peace as they responded in prayer to our needs.

When we gather at Tim and Becky's house Tim's dad Nick, who is 84, is usually sitting in the corner wing chair. He has grown bent with age and leans heavily on his walker when he stands to greet us. When he sees Wayne he always stretches his arms out for a hug. They have forged a bond of mutual affection and prayer between them, this Dutchman and Sicilian. Nick communicates God's love with a Mediterranean flair.

Another stress reliever I rediscovered could be initiated with a simple text message: "Got an hour for a cup of coffee." Just getting out of the house and meeting a friend or two at a coffee shop seemed to act as a steam valve lowering internal pressure.

*****

"They meet next Tuesday evening. Do you want to go?"

The elders at our church offer prayers and oil on the first Tuesday of each month. Although we had experienced the prayers of many faithful prayer warriors, we had not gone to the elders. We had not grown up in a church with this tradition, but James 5:14 says, *Is any one of you sick? He should call the elders of the church to pray over him and anoint him with oil in the name of the Lord.*

Meredith had asked us about it at just about the same time Wayne and I felt an urge to go. She wanted to come and so did Justin. On the first Tuesday in May, they met us at church at 7 o'clock.

Another new experience. Wayne paced a bit in the hall as we waited. Only a few minutes passed before we were called into the informal meeting room and greeted by four elders and a woman who coordinated the appointments. Smiles, introductions, a few "I recognize you." Then we sat in a circle.

"What moved you to come here tonight?" one of the elders asked.

"My wife."

Everyone laughed and the tension was gone.

Wayne explained what he had gone through in the past few months and that it looked like we were going back to Mayo Clinic soon.

"This is regular oil. I'll put a drop on your forehead. We'll pull the circle tighter. Come closer Meredith, Justin. And we'll pray."

Heads bowed, hands rested on Wayne's shoulders, holy moments flowed around us. The words that linger in my mind, "Lord, we pray boldly in Jesus name for Wayne. We pray for a miracle of healing that will astound his doctors and bring glory to Your name."

Tears sprang up, but peace and hope were nourished. How incredibly grateful I am for obedient elders, a receptive husband, and believing children. We were strengthened for whatever God had planned for us. *Thank you Father. You are faithful.*

Pondering

How do you spend special days like Easter and Christmas? Can you recall a season when news was disappointing and the weight of the moment was heavy? What acts of obedience have you felt called to? How did they bless you?

Chapter 17

Lite Brite, Curve Balls, and Boldness

Such confidence as this is ours through Christ before God. . . . Therefore, since we have such a hope, we are very bold. II Corinthians 3:4 and 12

"Grandma, I made a list of five things for us to do." My talkative five year old Ryan had carefully prepared for our time together when I came to babysit. The Lite Brite pegs were divided into two piles on the kitchen table, waiting for me. "You use that side, and I'll use this one."

My cell phone rang just as I picked up my first peg. "Oh, Ryan, I'm so sorry. I have to take this. It's Papa's doctor."

She lifted her fingers to her mouth, twisted her hand, and "locked" her lips.

It was Mayo Clinic. There was a problem with the insurance that had to be straightened out before we arrived there the following week. I copied down the information I needed, called the insurance company, and conveyed it to them and gave them the fax number for Mayo. Another call beeped in from Mayo as I finished that call. Twenty-five minutes later I was finally able to hang up.

"Done," I told Ryan. She unlocked her lips. She had not made a sound or moved off her chair for twenty-five minutes! What had come over her? Still quiet, she turned the Lite Brite around so I could see her design: a small red glowing heart with the words *I love you* in gold and white lights sparkling next to it.

For the remaining two hours we had together we played and did all the activities on her list. Enormous blessings in a pint-size package.

*****

We had received Wayne's Mayo appointment schedule in the middle of April for his trip back to Rochester in May. Finally, the fourth round of chemo was completed, the next one postponed, the insurance papers in order, and the car packed. A day or so before we left Stephanie and Meredith informed us that they would be flying out to join us for three days. They told us there was no point arguing since the tickets were purchased and non-refundable. Heart-strong daughters!

Had I packed enough, too much? How long would we be living out there? More questions than answers again. It was a grandchild's words that echoed in my mind as we pulled out of the driveway turning my thoughts from worries to gratitude.

The previous weekend we had gathered as a family to celebrate William's 7th birthday. The seed of enthusiasm for hockey planted at the Griffins' game in January had sprouted. He chose the Detroit Red Wings for his party theme. We had all dressed in red and white, and Aunt Meredith made one of her special cakes, this time a hockey rink. A hockey net was set up in the driveway and Uncle Paul provided hockey sticks and a ball that made a pretty good puck.

"You know what I love about this family?" I said to Aubrey as we sat and chatted the next day. "I love how everyone joins in to celebrate birthdays, like William's yesterday."

"I love how we support each other like when Uncle Justin got divorced, Papa got cancer, and when Mitchie (her beloved dog) died. That's what I love."

Five year olds, eight year olds can notice more than we realize. They make me think.

*****

Chicago traffic can be a challenge, we learned, at just about any time of the day. My cell phone rang as the cars and trucks around us seemed to be multiplying exponentially.

"Wayne's appointments have all been rescheduled for next week. I'll give you the new schedule."

Before a wave of despair could take root, God gave me clarity of mind and courage to say, "That's unacceptable. Wayne's treatment has been delayed so we could come this week. We are almost halfway there, and our daughters are flying in tomorrow. We've had this schedule for a month. You cannot change it now. If nothing else, please schedule the PET scan and a meeting with Dr. B. Please! We are not turning around."

"I'll see what I can do."

Wayne had slowed down and pulled into the right lane looking for an exit. "What's going on?"

"Keep going. They are saying all your appointments are changed to next week. We've got some praying to do."

Text message can trigger prayers, and they did that morning. Thirty minutes later Mayo called again. "Okay I think we can make this work. Here is your new schedule. Can you write it down?"

Grateful, I noted each of the appointments and then stopped. "Wait, you have the scan last. What good will the meetings do if the doctors don't have the scan?"

"Sorry, that's the best I can do. But maybe if you get here this afternoon they can fit you in."

Okay, we can do this. Nothing but stops to fill up the gas tank and run to the rest room. We arrived an hour before the deadline she had set. We scrambled to find the right building and office only to be told: "We don't take any more patients after 3:00 p.m." It was 4 o'clock.

Explaining our dilemma didn't change the policy, but she did offer this: "Maybe we can fit you in tomorrow morning. We start at 6:00 a.m."

"We'll be here."

"Oh, and you need blood work before that. The lab is downstairs. They open at 6:00 a.m."

5:45 the next morning we were third in line at the lab. We watched employees come in and at 6:05 Wayne's name was called for the blood work. At 6:15 his name was on the call list for the scan.

"We are booked solid, but you can wait until 9:00 a.m. You have your first appointment with the doctors at 10:30 so we can't take you in after 9:00."

Please God make a way.

I sent more text messages to family and friends, hoping that when they woke up they would see them and add their prayers to ours.

The waiting room filled up; names were called; new patients arrived to take the empty seats, and the clock ticked on.

Neither of us had eaten. Wayne needed to follow a low sugar diet before the scan, and had no appetite anyway. 6:30 . . . 7 . . . 7:30 . . . . Encouraging texts were coming in from family and friends assuring us of their prayers. At 7:50 a.m. I asked Wayne if he minded if I went for a cup of coffee.

"Go, please get yourself something to eat too. You know I'll be here when you get back, and if I'm not, well praise God, my name was called."

"I'll hurry."

8:05 I returned and could not find Wayne in the waiting room. His name had been called!

At 10:30 a.m. we met with the dermatologist who had removed the cyst. Kindness marked his demeanor. "I just received your scan. The oncologist will go over it with you in detail."

And, and . . . what do you see?

He smiled as he looked at Wayne, "The report does say 'nearly complete response to the treatment.' This is remarkable."

The next hour we met with Dr. H the radiologist. He also studied the scan and report and his enthusiasm could not be mistaken, "This is fantastic!"

Finally, we met with Dr. B the oncologist. "Wow! This is a wow."

Each time we praised God and verbally acknowledged, "God has done a great thing."

Would this be the end of Wayne's cancer fight? Were we almost finished?

"Well, while we see no sign of cancer, we still say 'nearly complete' because there are microscopic cancer cells that may be lurking." Dr. B was preparing us for his next suggestion for treatment. "I will consult with the other doctors and let you know what we think you should do. Meanwhile, you have a lot to be happy about. We'll talk again tomorrow."

"Doctor, we have a lot to praise God about. And we thank God for you. You are one of the answers to our prayers."

Bold prayers, confident actions, verbal testimony! All God-empowered.

*****

Late that afternoon we waited on the sidewalk. The girls had flown into Minneapolis and rented a car to drive to Rochester. The little white rental pulled up to the curb with windows down and two precious daughters waving.

"We got your text message when we landed. How did all this happen so fast? Looks like we came to celebrate! Yahoo!"

Pondering

Can you recall a moment or event in which a child surprised you with grace? –insight? Have you ever experienced a stubborn strength that you know must be God-inspired?

Have you ever experienced God's timing in every little detail of the day?

Chapter 18

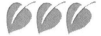

Celebrations, Ambush, and a Gentle Reminder

The Lord your God is with you, He is the Mighty Warrior who saves. He will take great delight in you; He will quiet you with His love; He will rejoice over you with singing. Zephaniah 3:17

Rochester is a welcoming city, geared for the thousands of patients who come from all over the world seeking help. The sidewalks around the Mayo buildings sparkle with inlaid glass, catching the sunlight. Each entry holds enormous pots of cascading flowers. Even along the side streets there are planters of greens with flowers of yellow, purple, and rose hues.

Before the girls had arrived, we had explored the area, walking, praising, and searching.

"That looks like a great place to go for supper with them." Wayne pointed to a restaurant on the corner, Victoria's. Perhaps it was the name that first caught his eye. It looked like just the right place to revel over the good news.

Two hours later we were settled in a booth by the window. The waitress noticed our high spirits, "Are you celebrating tonight?" We couldn't resist sharing. "God is so good, and I'm so happy for you. What would you like tonight?"

My cell phone rang as our meals arrived. Mayo. "Hello."

"I'm calling to tell you about your schedule next week."

What schedule???

Before I could ask she continued: "Dr. L (the surgeon) has Wayne scheduled for more surgery on the primary cancer site next Thursday at 8:00 a.m."

"Are you sure? Nobody said anything about that at our meetings today."

"I'm not sure, but that decision was probably made after the doctors reviewed the results. Please let us know by tomorrow if you can be here."

Wayne and the girls were chatting and eating. I picked up my fork, no longer hungry.

"What was that call, Mom?"

"They want Dad to come back next week for more surgery. We have to let them know by tomorrow morning, if we can come."

Gloom threatened to steal everyone's appetite. How do we recover some of our joy after that call? Was surgery really necessary?

"We have a meeting with Dr. B tomorrow morning to go over all the results. We'll see what he thinks."

"Okay, everybody. Lots of good stuff happened today. We'll worry about that tomorrow." Wayne's attitude shifted us all back in the right direction.

As we got up to leave, the waitress asked me if everything was alright. "Oh, the food and service were great! The phone call gave us a jolt. We may have to come back next week."

"May I ask your husband's first name? I would like to pray for him and your family." A stranger wanted to pray for us?! It would be months before we bumped into her again, but it was one of the many details we experienced that only God could orchestrate.

The girls had brought lots of treats with them and that night we played Sequence and cards and laughed and chose joy.

Early the next morning we met the girls for breakfast and then headed over to Wayne's appointment. Maybe he would just want Wayne to have that last round of chemo that was still on the schedule in Grand Rapids. We were to learn he had a lot more in mind than just that.

After greeting the girls with his usual warmth he introduced the surgeon, dermatologist, and nurse who also came into the small examination room. "Let's go over the progress you have made. Then we'll discuss the next steps I think you should consider."

He began with the first scan taken in January. With great detail he pointed out the areas where cancer was clearly visible in Wayne's body. Then he put up the latest scan and compared the two.

Our eyes were fixed on the screen, "Dr. L recommends more surgery. We will discuss that further and let you know."

I never breathe deeply until I am sure the doctor has nothing more to add. That time he did.

"I think you should come back to Mayo for five weeks of radiation. We can't see any signs of cancer, but we know there are microscopic cells. Your cancer was in a very sensitive area of the pelvis. Dr. J has been on my team for ten years specializing in pelvic radiation. Your chances of serious side effects from the radiation will be greatly reduced under his care."

He paused.

"Wayne, this is your decision. This is just my advice. Call me and let me know what you decide. We'll set up the appointments if you choose to come."

God is this part of the plan? Didn't you heal Wayne? Do you want us to come back? I can't believe it! 5 weeks! Where will we live? How can we do this? Where are you?

My anguish reminded me of a visit from my courageous niece Jami, who had also been on a rugged cancer journey of her own. The day before we left for this trip, she had stopped by to assure us of her love and prayers and to give us a nugget of wisdom that resonated. She said it carried her through difficult times, when the cancer journey looked like an insurmountable mountain and the path looked too high and steep. "Uncle Wayne, you have to be a threshing machine."

"Don't worry, God will make you one: *See I will make you into a threshing sledge, new and sharp, with many teeth. You will thresh the mountains and crush them, and reduce the hills to chaff. You will winnow them, the wind will pick them up, and a gale will blow them away. But you will rejoice in the Lord and glory in the Holy One of Israel.* Isaiah 41:15-16."

Meredith linked arms with Wayne as we stepped off the elevator, offering encouraging words. Stephanie and I walked behind them, silent, pondering. She leaned against a large column, and I paused. I heard it through the muffled conversations of hundreds of people in the large marble lobby. The sound reverberated off the walls. I couldn't see the piano or the gifted musician, but his music must have been chosen by my Father for that moment. The notes prompted the words to sing in my mind, "I sing because I'm happy. I sing because I'm free. For His eye is on the sparrow, and I know He's watching me."

Pondering

Have you ever felt like a threshing machine called and equipped by God to take on a mountain?

Chapter 19

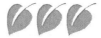

A Daughter's Heart

Stephanie: November 2016

I did not want to write this. I REALLY did not want to write this because the truth is I thought my dad was going to die and seeing those words in black and white type is very scary. It was much safer keeping that thought hidden in the back of my mind and pushed down to the bottom of my soul. But here is my attempt to express what the last year and half of cancer was like from my perspective.

From the beginning I had a bad feeling. Perhaps it's my personality. If you ask if I want the good news or bad news first, bad news first please, always. I like to know what I'm dealing with. Just the facts please Mama, don't sugar coat it, straight, no chaser. But as more details came in as doctors were trying to figure out what was wrong with my dad the news just went from bad to worse, and the knot in my stomach grew tighter and tighter.

When I first heard the diagnosis my mind immediately went to the Christmas before when Dad had been so sick with influenza. Had the cancer cells been doing their evil, destructive work even then, compromising his immune system? And then the word Merkel. What the What? The blessing and the curse of our modern day access to all knowledge "the internet" explained to me in great detail (much of which I did not understand) what Merkel cell carcinoma was. A cancer described as rare, aggressive and spreads quickly to other organs, all words I definitely understood, and the knot in my stomach squeezed tighter.

As the oldest daughter and a wife and a mother of three young girls, of course I wanted to be strong and helpful, for my parents, for my kids, for myself. But what could I do? Being two hours away and dealing with a little known cancer left me feeling very useless. Many cold, dark January nights, my sweet, loving husband would put the girls to bed and I would wash the dishes alone and weep. My sister Meredith and I talked about things in terms of "B.C." or before cancer. There was life before cancer which seemed relatively simple and then life after cancer, when most every waking moment is thinking about cancer and what it was doing to our family.

The first months of my dad's cancer diagnosis were full of confusion and heartbreak. Seeing my dad so overwhelmed and my mom so sad broke my heart. It was difficult for my dad to talk about it initially. I could see he needed to process the news, to just try and wrap his mind around how his world was just turned upside down. As a daughter, I still had a childlike picture of my dad as an invincible superhero. It was hard to watch him be vulnerable, poked and prodded, which I knew he hated and the constant questions, repeating the same information over and over again to different doctors all the while getting scarier and scarier insight into the cancer and the treatments that were on the road ahead.

With my stomach in knots and my mind racing "but what can I do?" I cried out to God, please. And He told me what I can do: Pray and Be. Call out honest, simple, gut-wrenching prayers, "Lord, heal my dad, Father God, strengthen my mom, Holy Spirit, please give us wisdom." I shared Dad's diagnosis with my women's Bible study and small group. They are a dedicated group of prayer warriors who offered up prayer, came alongside of me, and gave so much support. And I could be present when I was able. So we made more trips to Grand Rapids to just be together, have dinner, a hockey game, cry, and laugh.

I felt it was important for my kids to have an understanding of the seriousness of Papa's cancer so it was an open conversation, and they could ask any questions. We prayed for Papa every morning and every night. But it was a delicate balance, because I also did not want them to feel scared about the situation. Praying for Papa empowered them to do something, and being together with their cousins and aunts and uncles helped them know we were all in it together, loving, supporting, and fighting for Papa.

Through a series of miracles, my dad saw an oncologist at the Mayo Clinic in Minnesota who developed a treatment plan and Dad started chemotherapy in Grand Rapids the winter of 2015. In May 2015 my sister and I made a trip to Minnesota and met my parents at Mayo Clinic to meet with the doctors and discuss the next steps of Dad's treatment.

The next big prayer request was for wisdom to decide if surgery was necessary and where to have radiation done, Grand Rapids or Minnesota? Meredith and I wanted to be there to support my parents and also get firsthand information on pelvic floor radiation.

There is a moment sitting in a tiny exam room crowded in with Mom and Dad, my sister, the oncologist, surgeon, dermatologist and a nurse that stands out very clearly to me. The doctors were talking in their doctor voices and put an image of my dad's first scan from back in January up on a screen. I was looking at my dad's internal organs. I could see his heart and his lungs and his stomach, and there in the middle were huge, bright red blobs—cancer. I felt like all the air in the room had been sucked out and I couldn't breathe; my heart was in my throat, and my stomach fell to my knees. The doctors continued to talk, but I don't know what they were saying. What I knew in my mind to be a serious diagnosis of Merkel, I could now see with my very own eyes on a screen. Pounds of cancer spread all over his abdomen.

Then the next slide came up: no visible sign of bright red cancer shown. The immense gravity of the first slide and the amazing miracle of the second slide were overwhelming. After the meeting I remember standing in the massive lobby of the mighty Mayo Clinic. I leaned against one of the towering, cold marble columns and let the miracle of what I had witnessed wash over me. My eyes filled with tears, "Thank you God for the second slide!"

Chapter 20

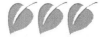

Sheepskin Confirmation

Have I not commanded you? Be strong and courageous. Do not be terrified; do not be discouraged, for the Lord your God will be with you wherever you go. Joshua 1:9

I felt like Gideon. Had we been given our marching orders? Wayne and I thanked God for the miracle of the excellent scan and the over-the-top support of our girls. But on the long ride home we also wondered what we should do next. What were God's plans?

Gideon's story is one of my favorites. Not because of his strength, but because of his doubts and need for confirmation. I can relate to that. His story is told in Judges 6 and 7. He was hiding out in a winepress threshing wheat, trying to save it from marauding enemies, when an angel of the Lord came and addressed him as *mighty warrior*. He then went on to tell Gideon his assignment: *You are going to save the Israelites from these enemies who oppress you.*

Gideon had plenty of excuses to get out of the assignment, basically they all came down to *I'm too weak—no "mighty warrior." Are you sure you mean me?*

God was patient and reassured Gideon by allowing him to put out a sheepskin overnight. Gideon wanted proof that he was hearing God's will correctly. The first time Gideon asked for the sheepskin to be dry in the morning, but the ground around it wet with dew. It was. The second time he asked for the sheepskin to be wet and the ground around it dry. It was. Gideon took the assignment and defeated the enemy.

Were we doubting God's healing power if we went? Were we avoiding a difficult, but necessary part of this journey if we refused to go? Would Wayne pay dearly later for not obeying now? How could we afford to go? How could we afford not to go? *Show us your plan Lord!*

The answers began to roll in on Sunday morning. Our pastor Jim Samra had begun a series on Joshua a brave leader who needed assurance that he was following God's plan and that God would lead the way. The verse and the message reminded us that *God will be with you wherever He has called you to go.*

Monday I met with a dear friend who was a palliative care nurse and had helped me understand medical issues. Barb had urged us to have chemo in Grand Rapids when we started, and I thought she would encourage us to stay home for treatment if Wayne got radiation. I was a bit stunned by her insistence that we should go to Mayo.

Another call came from Mayo that Monday, saying with further consideration they had decided the surgery on the original spot was not necessary. We could just come back for the five weeks of radiation. "Please let us know what you decide about that."

Tuesday at golf a friend I had not asked for insight pulled me aside to say, "I'm not sure why I'm telling you this, but you have to go back to Mayo for Wayne."

Tuesday night another dear friend, a nurse called to say she had been praying about us with a fellow nurse and both felt they needed to urge us to return to Mayo.

Wayne and I prayed for a voice of guidance, and God sent a chorus. Within a few days we had moved from doubt of what we should do, to unity among us and the family members that we had to go.

We did not know where we would stay, who would take care of things at home, how we would cover all the expenses, and if insurance would cooperate. We just knew we had to make a phone call and tell Mayo we were coming back.

*****

Before we could return for the five weeks of treatment, Dr. H., the radiologist, needed time to make a precise plan and a mold of Wayne's body which would hold him in place during the radiation procedure. So in the second week of June we drove again for the day of planning and mold making. I had checked online for a reasonably priced hotel close enough to walk to the appointments.

Sometimes you can't trust reviews. It was close; it did have a lobby; it did serve breakfast; but nobody had mentioned that it was depressing. This would not be a good *home-base* for the time we would need to stay.

Walking the neighborhood around Mayo gave us a better idea of what was available. We had been told about Hope Lodge, a wonderful place where long-term Mayo patients can stay—if there is room. Stopping there we learned that it would be a week or more after we arrived for our long stay before anything might open up. But, they did offer us a coupon good at a number of hotels which would cut the normal rate in half while we waited. What a gift of hospitality!

We walked over to the Kahler Inn and Suites directly across the street from the building where Wayne would have radiation five days a week. Being a bit suspicious of lobbies and reviews I asked if I could see a room and explained that we would need to stay for a week or longer before moving to Hope Lodge.

"Of course, let me show you a couple of options." Donald at the front desk was quick to smile and offer assistance. He showed us two rooms: first, a regular hotel room and second, a mini-suite. That could work! It included a small kitchen. I knew we would not want to go out for every meal, and the price with the Hope Lodge coupon was far less than we expected. We put in a reservation for the following week.

On the ride home I added to my list of what needed to be done before we went into exile. I wish I could say I was nothing but grateful, but that would be dishonest. *Exile* expressed how I really felt about going. I did not want to go. I knew we had to go. I believed God had patiently given the confirmation my sheepskin faith needed. But I hated trading the security and warmth of family and home for hotels and strangers. Michigan summers brought sunshine and more visits from my grandkids to play on the beach and jump off the dock, to grill outside and eat on the deck, to reconnect with my church golf buddies, to slow down and savor life. Most of the summer would be over when we returned, and how battered would Wayne be after this next assault on his body? The battle plan had all kinds of possibilities for collateral damage.

Trust and obey! That's what I kept repeating to myself as we checked off the to-do list. That old Sunday school hymn played over and over in my mind: *When we walk with the Lord in the light of His Word, what a glory He sheds on our way. When we do His good will, He abides with us still, and with all who will trust and obey. Trust and obey for there's no other way to be happy in Jesus, but to trust and obey.*

Thursday night Stephanie and Paul returned with the girls. Overcast skies surrounded us as we sat on the beach and watched the girls swim, but we felt the warmth of the sun and saw glimpses of its rays. Friday night the family met for food, laughter, and the gift of a small bag packed with cards they had made and written—one for each day we were to be gone. We would discover what a treasure-filled bag of love it was, giving us a link to home and food for our hearts.

Saturday night Nan and Jim invited us over with a group of friends for an impromptu pizza and prayer party. What holy moments as we sat in a circle and prayed for each other. Each one of us had experienced seasons of pain and knew the difference prayers made. We left there with hugs and a small tin with the words Prayer Box on the lid. It held papers on which our friends had written their prayers for us along with blank sheets for us to write ours.

Sunday we witnessed our Lauren "stand-up" to profess her faith in Jesus Christ at the morning service. Priceless moments we were so thankful to witness. Sunday afternoon we packed the car and answered the doorbell to a visit from Warren and Marybeth (Aunt Beth). Warren and Wayne are not only twins, they are also best friends. They share a unique closeness and affection. Marybeth and I have laughed about being glad we are also good friends, knowing we will probably never move very far away from each other. They gave Wayne a Life is Good tee-shirt. I saw the strain on Warren's face as he hugged his brother good-bye.

Lisa and Todd from our small group delivered a bag with a one-of-a-kind gift for each week we were gone. Lisa has a great sense of humor and that gift bag came with smiles in it.

Barb and Art also made a quick visit for a hug, a prayer, and precious words of encouragement.

Perhaps it was the distance, maybe the diagnosis, maybe the treatment he was facing; something triggered dear people to fill us with their gifts of love and prayers. They were the best things we loaded into the car.

Monday morning we left with the ticket our kids had given us to take the shortcut to Mayo on the Lake Express Ferry leaving from Muskegon. A thick fog blanketed Lake Michigan as we pulled out of the harbor. The journey in the next five weeks seemed to be hidden in an uncertain future, but like our trust in the boat captain, we trusted the One who was guiding our path.

Pondering

What helps you confirm the will of God? What gives you peace in the fog?

Chapter 21

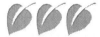

Unexpected News, Envelopes, and Dorm Life

Consider it pure joy, my brothers and sisters, whenever you face trials of many kinds, because you know that the testing of your faith develops perseverance. Let perseverance finish its work so that you may be mature and complete, not lacking anything. James 1:2-4

"It's a suggestion, but I think it would be wise." Dr. B settled back in his chair and waited.

At Wayne's first radiation appointment on the Monday afternoon we arrived, we had been given a new schedule. This one included a meeting with Dr. B on Tuesday morning that would rattle our spirits.

"More chemo? Stronger chemo? This isn't what I expected." Wayne's questions and face clearly expressed his disappointment.

"Why? Did you see more cancer?"

"No, but cancer cells can be invisible and return. I just think we should take every precaution to prevent that from happening. It's up to you."

Wayne looked at me. I could offer no advice. I was just trying to breathe. The chemo Dr. B recommended was powerful, and with that power there were multiple side effects possible. Could Wayne in his weakened state tolerate that AND the radiation? These "cures" seemed like loose cannons knocking out not only cancer cells. *Oh God, would I lose Wayne to the very things that were supposed to be helping him? What would be left of him after this?*

The next morning radiation was followed by the first long session of chemotherapy. Wayne had decided it was the right thing to do. He chose to have a good attitude about it and felt at peace after listening to Dr. B's research and reasons for the treatment. It took me longer to feel the peace he expressed.

Life felt unsettled, unreal as we woke up each morning in a hotel with only treatments on our calendar. We had to figure out how to live each day without sinking into despair. One activity we established took some discipline: opening the envelopes from home. There were times we just wanted to tear them all open. But each one had a number on it: Day 1, Day 2 . . . Day 15 . . . Day 20 . . . Day 30 . . . Last Day. So we established a routine: Make coffee, have devotions, open the envelope of the day—and only that one!

The first one was a homemade one-page calendar that began on June 14 and ended on July 17 the day we hoped to go home. Some days it was a handmade card of knock-knock jokes, sometimes a drawing, sometimes a store-bought card with a handwritten message, one time a pair of big bright blue socks for each of us—one pair marked I Love Grandma and one marked I Love Grandpa. Every member of the family contributed. One note included a Starbucks card. Ashlyn sent us a cross she had made in Sunday school to remind us Jesus loved us. William carefully drew each of the 50 states and labeled them—reminding us of the floor puzzle he loved to do at our house. He put Minnesota on the front page. The back page told us to *Read Psalm 23.*

How those pieces of paper and words ministered to us and both fed and eased our homesickness. We taped each one on our door and often caught each other rereading them. Don't ever underestimate the power of words and drawings and small gifts to speak of love and home. Another lesson my family taught me.

*****

"Let's go golfing!"

"Are you up to it?"

"Why do you think I tried to schedule all my treatments in the morning?"

We had brought our golf clubs, but they had remained unused in the car. We had walked the streets of Rochester, gone to treatments, and rested. The thought of getting-out-of-town felt really good. Wayne searched the internet for local golf courses. There were quite a few.

"Let's drive around today and check out the courses. We'll choose one to play tomorrow." Wayne handed me his list with the addresses.

This non-techie person that I am became increasingly grateful for GPS that navigated us out of town and through the countryside surrounding Rochester. As we found each one, Wayne liked to pick up a score card, talk to someone about the course, and walk to the first tee. I just relished the blue sky, the rolling hills, and a sense of normalcy.

Our final stop on the tour-of-courses brought us the farthest from town, past acres of grain stretching as far as I could see with farm houses visible in the distance, to a small sign with an arrow and the name of the golf course. There was no course in sight as we drove down a long winding dirt road.

I am so thankful we did not turn around. The course ended up being a place of sweet blessings.

We parked next to a few other cars in the lot and walked up to the small club house. Wayne headed straight for the restroom. That stent never gave him a break for very long. The woman behind the counter greeted me, "What can I do for you?"

I explained that we were looking at golf courses and asked for a card.

"Are you new in the area?"

"Yes, just here for five weeks."

"At Mayo?" She had seen Wayne's appearance and his tell-tale bald head.

I nodded.

"Would you like to grab a golf cart out of the garage and take a drive around the course? I have a league starting in an hour, but you have plenty of time to see if you would like to come back and play."

Wayne was a bit stunned when he returned, and I explained her offer. Courses don't do that.

"What do I owe you for the cart?"

"Nothing, enjoy your ride."

Remember when you got your driver's license and got to take the car for the first time? That's what it felt like to be out on that bumpy cart! As we came up to the fourth hole we rode over a bridge crossing a shallow bubbling stream, and came through a woods filled with the sweet scent of pine. Suddenly we saw granite cliffs bordering the course.

A sense of God's presence filled us. We were facing mountains, but God had lovely valleys where He would provide rest. He would lead us by the still water and restore our souls for the work of threshing that lay ahead. He would reveal Himself and His provision through the kindness of people He brought into our journey. We would return to that course for more unexpected blessings in the weeks ahead.

An hour later my cell phone rang as we waited for our supper in a local restaurant back in town.

"Hello, this is Hope Lodge. We have a room ready for you. When may we expect you?"

"Can I call you back in a few minutes?"

We had been at the Kahler Inn for almost a week and were feeling settled, but I knew we had to do this: move again.

"Let's wait until tomorrow."

Saturday felt a little like moving into the dorms at Calvin College as a freshman. Up to the third floor, one room, a bathroom, television across the hall in a community room, kitchen on the first floor. Moving into that new adventure in the '60's was an easier adjustment than moving into this in our 60's. But Jennie knew that. She was one of the resident directors and had greeted us with kindness, gave us our keys, and explained that most of the people were gone for the weekend. She offered her prayers and assurance, "This will be a good place for you."

To be honest, I did not feel that . . . at first.

Waking up Sunday morning, Father's Day, after a week of treatments found Wayne very quiet, and his lack of banter and morning smiles added to my sadness, my loneliness. You might think that I should have been nothing but grateful to be able to be at Mayo, to have come this far in the cancer journey, to have experienced God's blessings in so many ways. But the truth is that maintaining a sense of gratitude, peace, and joy are a daily struggle and some days are harder than others. This was a hard one.

Learning that choosing joy was a decision I needed to make every day had helped me through days of discouragement and brokenness in the past. It's not easy. But it is so much better than sinking further into that awful swamp of despair. Joy is a gift from God. I discovered the Bible is full of verses about joy often referenced with suffering. I began to intentionally save them after I discovered Joyce Meyer about fifteen years ago.

I found her program *Enjoying Everyday Life* while I sipped my early morning coffee, trying to wake up before school. She became my *spiritual chiropractor* adjusting my attitude from *poor-tired-me* to *I can do all things through Christ who strengthens me* (Philippians 4:13). I bought her bestseller *Battlefields of the Mind* and learned important lessons about choosing what I would think about, how to live by faith and not just by feelings, and how to focus on His strength, not my weakness.

Years later I downloaded her app on my phone and that morning I listened and took in truths I knew, but needed to put front and center in my thinking.

"Let's go find a fun local breakfast place and take a walk," I suggested. Thankfully, Wayne agreed. We found Jennie by the desk and asked where she would go.

"If you are up for a walk, I would suggest my favorite place, Cheap Charlie's. It's popular with locals so it might be busy."

Fifteen minutes later we spotted the huge plastic hog sitting on the flat roof above the sign: Cheap Charlie's. She was right, it was busy. It had delicious food and the charm of dated tiles, plastic red cups, and an open view to the kitchen behind the counter.

I shared our day on a Facebook post: *Week One at Mayo completed! 6 radiation treatments, 5 chemo treatments, 2 moves, one 404 miles from Grandville to Rochester and the second 3 blocks from the Kahler Inn to Hope Lodge, at least 2 dozen cheerful Mayo nurses and staff, a few homesick tears and moments of discouragement, countless prayers, and one awesome God who never let us go. So we celebrate Father's Day for the first time in 4 decades without any of our kids. We still celebrate because we have a Heavenly Father who is taking care of all His children. Blessings to all earthly dads who have shared the love of Jesus from generation to generation.*

Pondering

Have you ever had to adjust to a new living situation? Can you recall what helped? How can time outside either taking a drive or a walk be refreshing?

Chapter 22

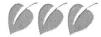

Lemons and Orange Juice

Though the fig tree does not bud and there are no grapes on the vines . . . yet I will rejoice in the Lord, I will be joyful in God my Savior. The Sovereign Lord is my strength, He makes my feet like the feet of a deer; He enables me to tread on the heights. Habakkuk 3:17-19

Goose poop had covered the beach the night before we left for Rochester. Leah and Jordan would be moving in a week after we left and the thought of William and Ryan playing on that sand drove me to a pail and shovel to clean up the mess—again! Those geese had been a pestilence and plague for the past month and in the morning they would be gently herded by a licensed company that would carry them to a wetland far from us!

Jordan and Leah's house had sold in less than a day a few weeks earlier, but they hadn't found a new place yet. We had asked them if they would like to stay with us. They planned to move in while we were gone. I was so glad they got to enjoy our little beach and lake during the summer months. William and Ryan were excited.

Leah told me later that the beach was clean when they arrived—small victory. She also shared with me: *I was relieved that critical treatment was being done at Mayo itself. My own little family was going through the transitional time of moving and all the emotions that go along with that. We needed to be out of the house we had sold and had no idea where God was going to land us long term. It just felt right to move into your home. I had much peace about it, and it was such an adventure for the kids!*

It was a blessing you were gone during this time because it was crazy and overwhelming having our stuff all over your house. It gave me time to organize and minimize the impact for when you would come home. The family continued to pull together while you were gone. We had get-togethers and parties while you were away, upholding the traditions you had started. We knew our bond would be a blessing to you. Your absence was always felt, but it was a joy to see the texts and pictures of you and Dad making the best of your time in Minnesota.

We wanted everyone to savor the summer; it's so brief and seems to fly by—usually. The passing of time in Rochester had changed for us, slowed down, dragged. It did not have wings; it seemed to have weights. At times twenty-four hours felt more like seventy-two. We had to make more of an effort to push through long mornings, afternoons, and evenings. Looking back, I realize we were adjusting to the physical, emotional, and social challenges we were facing. I am thankful we made an effort to start the day asking for direction and then making ourselves get out, walk, do something.

Mayo Clinic has a long history of recognizing the need for music, beauty, art, education, and encouragement to strengthen the mind and the body and the spirit. Some of the gifts to patients and their families that I especially appreciated were the grand pianos found in various buildings. Anyone was welcome to stop a while and play or listen.

Wayne's radiation treatment usually took about a half hour. I would wait with him until his red beeper called him from the waiting room to a restricted area. Sometimes I would journal, or try to read, but what helped me the most was going to the piano in the nearby lobby and quietly playing hymns or classical music.

If I saw a patient near the piano, I would ask if they minded if I played. One time a man looked up from his book and answered my question with, "Not if you're good." Bit of pressure, but I played a few songs anyway, and when I left he smiled, "That was good."

Mayo often had guests performing in the lobbies. We learned to check the schedule and attended quite a few recitals of singers, bands, string quartets. We also took an art tour led by a retired Mayo doctor and were astounded to learn about the many famous artists who have donated work to Mayo. The subway halls that wind under the streets and buildings of the clinic providing protection from inclement weather are lined with beauty.

Two weeks had passed and the 4th of July was approaching, one of our favorite days of the year. When we moved to Grandville we discovered that we were only a few blocks from the town's all-out patriotic parade. Residents start gathering at 6:00 a.m. to put their blankets and chairs in their favorite spots. When my Mom came to Michigan at the age of 93 and was living with us, I had pushed her wheelchair up to a crowd at least six people deep. They opened a spot for her and the people nearby grabbed the necklaces and small balls that were tossed from the floats before they could accidently hit her. I knew we had moved to a good place.

As the grandchildren grew I began a tradition of buying them matching 4th of July tee shirts. Stephanie and Paul would come to town for several days. Stephanie, Meredith, and Leah became artists, face painting flags, stars, and rainbows on smiling little cheeks. Papa would hand out small flags just before we made our own parade of red, white, and blue marching down to the spot I had saved with quilts early that morning.

At night Justin put on the best-ever fireworks display over the lake that ended when the Grandville fireworks could be seen lighting up the sky. Family, friends, neighbors would join us for supper and the show, bringing a chair and a dish to pass. Babies watched with their mamas from the family room windows, wheelchairs sat on the deck, canvas chairs of red and blue dotted the lawn. It was a really special time.

This year we would be in a nearly empty dorm, in a nearly empty city. July 3 was a Friday but Wayne had no treatments to give staff a much deserved 3-day weekend. We—maybe it was just I—thought of going home for the weekend. But we knew driving around Chicago on a holiday weekend was a bad idea. I knew the eight or nine hour trip each way would be too much. Wayne was tired. All the treatments were taking their pounds of flesh. It was only the third week of June.

Just when the anticipation of missing out on the memory-making weekend was getting me down we got a phone call from Stephanie.

"Mom, I have tickets for the girls and me to fly to Minneapolis on Tuesday. Can you pick us up?"

I had warned the family that their dad wasn't up for a lot of activity, that visiting would not be much fun, that summer was short, but that hadn't stopped them. They had plotted and planned to have three of them come out for two or three days, spaced over the time we were gone. Stephanie was to come first, alone, but Grace, Aubrey, and Ashlyn had pleaded to come, knowing it wouldn't be a vacation.

The sight of them coming through the gate at the airport was a shot of pure joy. I snapped a picture and they laughed, "You make us feel like movie stars, Grandma."

"You are to me—the best stars ever! Papa can't wait to see you."

Since the world-famous Mall of America is only ten minutes from the airport I thought we could stop there and at least this would be entertaining for them. We did stop, but not for long, even the amusement park did not hold the draw of seeing Papa. It wasn't long before we were back in the car for the hour drive to Rochester.

"We'll do something special. I'm usually done by 10:00 a.m.," Wayne promised the girls at breakfast the next morning. That day would not be usual.

"You're next, but something happened to the computer system. It may take only a few minutes to fix. You should wait."

One hour passed, then another. I had taken the girls to see some of the artwork in the subway, but they refused to go very far. Ashlyn is the youngest, bubbly on the soccer field, full of energy, and always on the go. She sat next to her Papa and seemed to need to simply rest against him. Who was this tender, quiet angel? For the third hour of waiting the girls sat close to Papa and talked. The waiting room had filled to overflowing with patients and family . . . waiting.

"You know what you do when life hands you lemons, Papa?" Grace asked somewhere in the third hour.

"Make lemonade?"

"Nope! Make orange juice and let people wonder how God did that!"

I've never forgotten the wisdom she shared. It's one of those funny things that sticks and comes back to me when life is feeling tart and bitter. I've learned to wait for the taste of sweet juice. Stephanie and her girls delivered the sweetness we needed—God gifts!

Finally a staff person announced, "Everything is fixed, so we can begin again." Wayne's red beeper lit up. He was the first one called.

What I did not know about was the emotional morning trip Stephanie made to rent a car the next day. Much later she shared with me the memories she titled:

Miracles in Minnesota

So often we have no idea what we really need. We pray in big, general terms or ask what we think we need to improve our situation, but thankfully God is a God of details and knows us intimately and gives us exactly what we need, when we need it. There were many miracles in Minnesota as I reflect on that time, amazing ways God showed up in small things that made a giant impact. I had no idea what I really needed, until God gave me exactly what I needed most.

Grace, Aubrey, and Ashlyn were excited to see Papa and Grandma when we went to visit my parents in Rochester. They were happy simply hanging out with them, swimming in the hotel pool, going out to eat, and accompanying Papa to his appointments. They spent hours in the waiting room sitting with so many people who had cancer, waiting for Papa's radiation treatment. They played silly games with him and listened to Grandma play the piano in the lobby. But just like the fun-loving, silly Dad, I remember as a child, he wanted the girls to do something fun on their "vacation" to Minnesota, despite the fact that he was receiving daily radiation and massive doses of chemo therapy during the fight of his life.

In the lobby of the hotel was the usual rack of brochures describing touristy things to do in the area. My dad found a brochure about caves we could visit and tour not too far from Rochester. I could tell it was important to him to do something different and show the girls a good time, so we decided to plan a road trip to a cave about an hour away.

The problem was my parents' five-passenger car did not fit the six of us. I called the local rental car company and spoke with a very friendly person on the phone. (I must say that every single person we came into contact with at the hotel, restaurants, Hope Lodge, and Mayo Clinic were beyond friendly and helpful. Rochester, MN is one nice town.)

I explained that I wanted to rent a car the next day and was hoping they had a six-passenger vehicle available. The alternative was to rent a small, economy car and drive separately, but my gut was telling me we needed to be together. The gentleman on the phone said unfortunately there were no minivans available. They did have a few SUV's, but he did not know if any had a third row.

The next morning the girls and I walked to the rental car company while Mom went with Dad for his morning radiation. It was a beautiful sunny day, perfect for a road trip out of town, but I started to feel nervous. We really needed to drive together. What if they didn't have a car we all fit in?

The friendly twenty-something year old man behind the rental counter said he would be happy to drive us over to the parking structure to check out the SUV. As we rode there he told us about all the people he had met from around the world who came to Mayo for treatment. I was only half listening when I started to silently pray, "Please God, I know we've asked a lot of you during this cancer journey. I know this is kind of silly. I know in the scheme of life this is a small thing. But please, we really need a car that holds all of us. Please God, give us a car with a third row."

We circled our way up the floors of the garage, finally stopping behind an SUV. He got out, unlocked it, and popped the back. "Oh, yeah," he said casually. "It has a third row."

I don't know if any rental car employee in the world has ever seen someone so excited to find out a car has a third row. I let out a few hoots, hoots with fist pumps, and high-fived the girls. They were happy and hooting too, though I'm sure they didn't quite know why. Then, I hugged the rental car guy much to his surprise and to my daughters' embarrassment.

My dad ALWAYS drove on our family vacations when I was a kid, so, feeling like a kid again, I asked if he wanted to drive. He smiled and softly said, "No doll, it's okay; you drive."

The girls chatted away with Grandma in the back of the car as we headed south out of Rochester. Dad looked especially thin and frail in the passenger seat of the car. His physical decline had initially seemed gradual to me, and he was always putting on a good face, but in that moment he looked very sick, but also very peaceful.

We rolled down the windows as the city gave way to country. The quiet two-lane road went through farm country and over rolling hills. Sometimes life can feel like a movie and that was one of those distinct, surreal times. We listened to music as we drove, the soundtrack to our life, some of Dad's favorite bands including Trampled by Turtles and Mumford and Sons.

We stopped at all the "scenic views" along the way and took pictures. We laughed and chatted. We found the cave, but the girls preferred mining for "gems" in a small water trough outside. We had a picnic under a shady tree and did all the other touristy things like play putt-putt and buy souvenir rocks in the middle of nowhere in Minnesota. And it was perfect, exactly what we needed.

Thank you, God, for that third row.

Time had wings while we went on a road trip, walked the sparkly sidewalks of Rochester, ate together at Hope Lodge. They delivered love, laughter, and home in every moment we spent with them. And all too quickly it was time to leave again for Minneapolis. We could fit only five in the car, and Wayne needed to go for a radiation treatment, so I would drive Stephanie and the girls back.

We lifted their suitcases into the car, the girls hugged Papa and jumped in, and then Stephanie reached for her dad. Arms tightened, eyes blinked hard, and they held on to each other for that extra lingering moment. "Go," he whispered to me, "get going." He was struggling.

One hour later I parked in the Minneapolis Airport parking garage, and Stephanie's phone beeped with a message, "Your flight has been canceled today."

Ordinarily, that would have been cause for rejoicing, but they were eager to get home. Paul was leaving for a rare overseas business trip, and they wanted to see him before he left. As reluctant as I was to see them go, I wanted them home for him.

"Let's see if there are any other flights today," Stephanie calmly encouraged the girls and began making phone calls as we walked to the desk.

"Okay girls, come with me while your mom works on flights. Let's go check out the toy store, and you can show me ideas for Christmas presents." The girls kept one eye out for their mom as they half-heartedly looked at the merchandise.

"Looks like we got some more lemons, Grandma," Grace said.

"Yes, and I wonder what kind of juice will come from this."

Ashlyn had seemed to be the most upset about the delay, but suddenly smiled. "This, Grandma, I want this!"

"What is it?" She handed me a stuffed toy totally yellow, with one enormous eye, wearing a pair of blue jean overalls.

"Grandma, don't you know *minions*?"

By the time Stephanie returned the girls had given me a fairly comprehensive education about the movie *Despicable Me* and the memorable minions.

"There's nothing until tomorrow. I called the Kahler Inn again, and they have our room waiting for us. I'll call Dad and let him know. We fly out early tomorrow morning and should be home in time to see Paul before he leaves."

The second time Wayne and Stephanie said goodbye was a little easier.

*****

Time returned to the tediously slow moments that had to be consciously passed. Later, when we returned home people would mention how quickly the weeks had flown while we were gone. It was another lesson to me that perception depends on a person's circumstances. Time is elastic. Never presume.

Thursday, July 2 we watched the grand exit from the city. Friday was quiet. Saturday morning began at 4:00 a.m. with a nightmare.

"I dreamt that I couldn't eat anything." Wayne had jerked awake from his dream. He had been having trouble chewing and swallowing for the last few days. The medication to relieve the pressure from his stent had been increased and the result was dry mouth. The chemo and radiation had already stolen most of his taste buds and his desire to eat, so dry mouth seemed like the final push to malnutrition.

God, please! He has lost so much weight. What can I do to help? Give me some ideas! Bring him relief. I felt a sense of panic and despair. It was still the holiday weekend, but we had to do something. He would see his doctor Tuesday morning. But what could we do now?!

Then I remembered a commercial for a product we had never needed before, Biotene, that Wayne could use to spray his mouth. Several hours later we found some at the pharmacy nearby. I went on-line to look up "dry-mouth" and ways to relieve it. When in a state of fear, even obvious things don't seem so obvious. Of course! He needed "wet food," things like soup and shakes. And he needed to cut back on the medication. The doctor had only suggested increasing it when Wayne expressed frustration with the frequent urgency the stent caused when he moved.

Our spirits were low. Waves of homesickness washed over us. I longed for a pair of Dorothy's ruby slippers that I could click as I thought, *There's no place like home.*

But God said, "Bloom where you're planted." So that's what we tried to do. By noontime Wayne experienced some relief. We took a long walk in the afternoon and then sat at an outdoor café surrounded by flowers. It helped. The home-front had been texting pictures of the face-painted grandkids sitting at the parade. Leah had gotten up early to go save seats in our favorite spot.

Justin shared with me: *Five weeks initially sounded like a long time to be gone, but when I really thought about it, it was nothing when I believed it would add years to having my dad in my life. The one night that it felt different for me was the 4th of July. Celebrating our annual party at your house without you there felt off. I enjoy putting on the fireworks show for the family, but the whole family wasn't there. I was very happy when we facetimed the fireworks. For a few minutes it felt right—we were all together.*

I knew I needed another attitude adjustment. Sunday morning it arrived via the computer. Calvarygr.org brought us back to our home church. Pastor Jim was preaching a series on Joshua. That morning he preached on Joshua 1:10-18. The tribes of Israel were finally going into the promised-land. Two and a half of the twelve tribes had received choice land east of the Jordan. They were set. But, they were still called to cross the Jordan and help everyone else. Jim reminded us to "live the story." When I am blessed—it's not just to sit back, but to see who needs my help. He pointedly said, "If you have gotten through cancer, see if you can help someone else on that journey."

More than an attitude adjustment, it was a wake-up call. Neither Wayne nor I said anything. He went down to the kitchen to start breakfast. When I came down a few minutes later, he was chatting with another Hope Lodge resident who was also battling cancer. That was the beginning. In the days and weeks ahead we got to know many residents, listened to their stories, were encouraged, and offered encouragement and our prayers.

Pondering

Have you noticed the elasticity of time? Can you recall a bitter experience that God infused with sweetness? Have you ever experienced an attitude adjustment that led to blessings?

Chapter 23

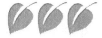

A Time for Everything: Enduring and Celebrating

There is a time for everything, and a season for every activity under heaven. . . . He has made everything beautiful in His time." Ecclesiastes 3:1 & 11

Wouldn't it be nice to just get through low times and begin a steady trajectory upward? We seemed to experience more of a step forward, two steps back, three forward, two back. Every day there were a least one or two skirmishes with despair.

We had improved Monday, thankful to have made it through the weekend. But Tuesday morning began on the edge of tears. Even devotions were difficult. God used a five year old to lift us up that morning. Each grandchild had contributed to the bag of cards. That morning we opened Ryan's. It was perfect—don't ask me why, but it did produce some smiles. "Why do cows wear bells? Because their horns don't work!" She hadn't signed it, but we recognized her crayon art and her large, bold printing.

Waiting for Wayne during his radiation that morning, I wrote in my journal: *There's always such relief when he walks out. My constant prayer: Please protect him from the side effects of radiation and destroy the cancer. I thought God would use me more directly out here, but as usual, His thoughts and purpose take me a while to discern. My key purpose is being here for Wayne. Wayne actually suggested I go home for a break. The thought of being away from him gives me chills. We both realize neither of us would do well.*

Occasionally I play the piano—that blesses me, but I've learned that it blesses others as well. A number of people have stopped to tell me. What seemed like a selfish action—to ease my soul—actually is used by God. So thankful.

As I sit here I see so many stages of suffering go by. Some faces strained, sad, resigned, but some peaceful, hopeful, still smiling. The greatest moment of pure joy is the moment someone rings the brass bell signifying the end of their radiation treatments. Everyone claps, not just the family surrounding them, everyone in the waiting room.

After radiation Wayne wanted to take a ride, anywhere. Noticing the tank was near empty we looked for a gas station and pulled into the Costco lot to fill up.

"Let's go in and walk around," Wayne suggested. "We can't buy anything, there's no room to put it, but we can look."

Odd how saying sure to that led to a much improved mood.

First, being there felt a little like home. We have a Costco in Grandville. Then we tasted some samples which led to buying a frozen lasagna. We only had two shelves in our community refrigerator and one freezer shelf, but, there was a potluck that night at Hope Lodge and we could bake this and choose to go—for the first time. This was the third way we were so blessed—in the going. But there was a second factor that improved our mood even before we walked out of Costco. We stopped to buy two frozen yogurts at the café, one strawberry and one twist. Grace in small things, even a frozen cup.

The hallway by the community dining rooms was lined with long tables filled with food. I added our offering to the hot foods and looked around for Wayne. He was talking with a tall, broad-shouldered man about our age. Later Wayne told me Joe had introduced himself after he noticed the golf logo on Wayne's shirt. Soon they discovered they had a mutual love for the game; they were both battling cancer; and they both had a wife named Elaine. Joe asked one more question that clinched a bond, "Do we have one more thing in common: Are you a man of faith?" Grace was part of the menu that night.

*****

Wayne insisted he felt fine, but I saw the belt holes, old ones bypassed for new ones needed to hold his loose pants, food pushed around his plate, naps, more frequent and longer, and a quietness that settled around him. He was still able to offer a smile and make someone chuckle when he went for treatments. I remember hearing the receptionists laugh out loud one day when he signed in. "What did you say to them?" I asked when he came to sit next to me in the waiting room.

"Oh, I told them I wasn't available."

"What?"

"They were talking about a friend who was looking for a husband. When they finally looked up at me, I told them 'Sorry, I'm not available.'"

Glimpses of the "old Wayne."

We found Meredith waiting for us at 8:15 a.m. two days later at the airport. Her flight had landed fifteen minutes earlier than expected. We breathed in her smiles and hugs like oxygen-deprived patients. She changed the color of the day, brightened it. We headed for breakfast to Canadian Honkers. For some reason people in Rochester love the very geese we try to chase off our lake and even name restaurants after them.

This cancer journey was wearing on both Wayne and me. Meredith's presence offered me a reprieve that I remember vividly. In the afternoon we decided to walk to the 1st Street Fair. It was warm and Wayne had left his hat in the car back at Hope Lodge several blocks away. Chemo makes skin burn easily, so he needed that hat. Meredith said she would go get it.

"No, I can. I forgot it." Wayne started walking back.

I just about grabbed the keys out of his hand and took off. It was strange, but I just felt an intense need to walk briskly, alone for a few minutes. It jarred Wayne to walk, pounding the stent, so our walks were unhurried, simply ambling, sometimes, at a snail's pace. For just a few minutes it felt good to be quick, efficient, business-like. Then I returned, content. I could only feel free to do that because Meredith was there.

Meredith brought her love, her easy chatter, and a renewed awareness of God's presence. I recall with gratitude being on a nearby lake with Meredith in a little electric paddle boat. A gentle breeze was blowing. Water lapped on the sides of the boat. I sensed God's Spirit whispering "I am with you." Healing moments when the crushing reality of cancer treatments eased.

I texted her after we reluctantly brought her back to the airport, *How do we say thank you for all the love and goodness you pour into our lives? Thank you! We love you.*

Her reply reflected her spirit, *I feel like I just showed up, and we walked and ate well. Easy! You both have the hard part.*

I knew it had not been easy making arrangements to come, leaving her family, missing work. But she did it with love and delivered joy to us.

*****

Wayne had finished another round of chemo. He had five more radiation treatments on the schedule. I dared to think about going home, but knew enough about the unexpected curves of this journey to wait before getting too excited. We had an appointment with Dr. B on Tuesday and knew he might suggest one more round. Wayne had lost a lot of weight and his muscle tone was declining. His smile was there, but his appearance had altered dramatically since our arrival.

We had texted pictures home, but I knew that actually seeing the impact of the treatments on their dad in person was hard on our kids. Wayne knew he could not hide the change.

Sunday night we drove together to Minneapolis. Jordan had informed us he wanted to come. No point arguing. We had learned that much. As we waited, Wayne asked for a piece of paper and a pen. He began coloring a large B on the paper. "What are you up to?" I asked.

"Just wait." Soon he held up a sign that read BUSH which he held against his chest as Jordan emerged through the sliding doors. It got exactly the response he wanted, a big grin on Jordan's face.

Summer heat was pounding Rochester. After radiation in the morning Wayne wanted to go golfing with Jordan. The temperature was climbing to 90. "Don't worry Mom, I'll make sure Dad drinks lots of fluids."

"I want to go back to that special course to thank them," Wayne added.

I knew which one he meant. I thought of it as the Psalm 23 course, a place of blessings. It was the course we had found on the "Tour of Courses" we went on during our first week in Rochester. The course where we had been given a golf cart to take a ride.

We had returned there a few weeks later to play nine holes. Again Wayne headed for the men's room when we arrived. I went to pay for nine holes and a cart. She wouldn't take my money.

"The owner says that anyone going through cancer treatment is going through enough. Golf is free. We can do that for you."

Tears surfaced at this unexpected kindness. Kindness can do that.

Wayne wanted to pay for a round with Jordan and just let them know how much that had meant to him. They left in high spirits. Later I learned they still wouldn't take Wayne's money and seven holes had been enough that day.

Our room was so quiet. It was the longest stretch Wayne and I had been apart since we had arrived. I sat and wrote again, recording the thoughts and events I would one day share.

Dr. H., Wayne's radiologist, had told Wayne that he had tolerated all the treatments exceptionally well and he would be done Friday. Would we be able to go home? We would find out on Tuesday when we met with Dr. B.

Monday night we decided to return to Victoria's, the restaurant we had gone to with Stephanie and Meredith in May when we were celebrating a great scan—before we knew about the advice to return for five weeks. That's where our waitress Jennifer had said she would pray for Wayne. It was a good place to celebrate with Jordan. When our waitress greeted us, was it a coincidence that it was Jennifer?

Tuesday morning Jordan went with us to Wayne's appointment with Dr. B. Had it been six months since we had first sat in this waiting room? It felt much longer. We had learned so much, been tested, and stretched. We braced ourselves for the news that more chemo might be needed, keeping us in Rochester longer. Wayne had described this city to a friend as "the beautiful city I never want to see again."

Dr. B got right to the point, "I can see no advantages to another round of chemo. You've taken everything we've thrown at you so well. You are a Poster Child. It's time to rebuild."

That deep breath of joy. I could see Wayne's eyes fill. "I was prepared to accept your recommendation for more chemo, but I did not want it."

Finally, we could make plans to go home!

Friday Wayne rang the brass bell after his final radiation. The car was packed and ready to go. As we pulled out of the harbor from Milwaukee a few hours later the sky was blue, the lake calm, and this time there was no fog, only a glorious sky as the sun set.

Pondering

Can you recall small choices, small pleasures that lifted despair during times of endurance?

Chapter 24

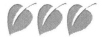

He Restores my Soul

Though you have made me see troubles, many and bitter, you will restore my life again . . . and comfort me. Psalm 71:20-21

It was after midnight before we finally pulled into our driveway. We had given the garage door openers to Jordan and Leah, so we stood on the front porch, like guests, and quietly knocked, not wanting to disturb William and Ryan. The door flew open at the first tap and we saw a glittering sign *Welcome Home.* We learned two eager grandchildren had made it that very afternoon. They were sleeping, but Jordan, Leah, and Justin were waiting.

The sight of them, their hugs, their joy, the reality of being home began the healing of deep weariness that afflicted Wayne, and I admit, me. It was after 1:00 a.m. when we finally said good-night, but when I opened my eyes at 6:00 a.m., Wayne was already up. I couldn't find him in the house, but had an urge to open the front door and simply see the familiar neighborhood. He was sitting on the white rocker, watching the sunrise. "I had to get up and thank God for . . ." He lifted his hand. The early morning light glistened on his tears.

Our small front porch became one of Wayne's favorite places. He sat with his morning coffee and devotions and greeted our walking neighbors. It became a place of fellowship. A place to say thank you to God and the dear neighbors who had prayed, cut the grass, raked the beach, edged the sidewalk, and welcomed us home.

Our family trip to Boyne Mountain was scheduled for the next week. While the grandkids simply delighted in having Papa back, or so I thought, the kids saw how much thinner and weary their dad was. They said, "Let's give Dad another week to get stronger." A call was made to Boyne and amazingly it was possible to reschedule with the same accommodations.

The scars from Wayne's battle with cancer and its treatments were evident. Food did not taste the same; his appetite was diminished; his muscle tone was gone. He knew he needed protein to rebuild. Leah helped me in our search for tasty, nutritious food. We tried smoothies, lots of fruits, and vegetables. Little by little we saw improvement.

The stent still plagued his movement, but Wayne never mentioned it. I knew by the way he moved and the occasional grimace on his face. August 12 was the next trip to St. Mary's for either removal or replacement of the stent. But that was several weeks away.

Meanwhile, we savored Michigan summer at its best, which meant lots of family time. It was the best time of year to have Jordan, Leah, Ryan, and William living with us as they looked for a house. If seven year old William wasn't jumping off the dock, he had a baseball glove on one hand, a ball in the other, and a bat close by. He wouldn't say much, just look at his Papa, waiting, hoping. Wayne spent hours not only passing, catching, pitching, but most importantly calling the game. "William hits one deep to left . . . . He rounds second, slides into third . . . . safe!"

One day as we played on the beach, Wayne went in the house. "Grandma, is Papa's cancer gone?" William had stopped playing to stand by me.

"Yes." My heart ached as I saw the hope and fear in his eyes.

"How? Like it's smashed?" He stomped his foot on the sand. I nodded.

He repeated the stomping, then picked up the sand and threw it into the water. Triumphant, he grinned, "Gone like this!" And we watched the sand disappear into the lake.

Finally, it was time to pack the car for fun, this time for four days of family vacation at Boyne Mountain. Four cars were packed with suitcases, food, golf clubs, and where they could fit—car seats and kids! Text messages flew from both sides of the state. Stephanie claimed, "Our bumper is dragging, but we'll beat you there!"

Seventeen of us gathered in the spacious lobby, giddy with excitement. Rooms weren't ready yet, but we could go to the water park. It seemed like life couldn't be any sweeter and then Jordan made an announcement. I had seen him take a call and step outside to talk. I noticed the grin on his face when he returned. He pulled Leah aside. She whooped and threw her arms around him.

Now we were all watching, waiting.

Jordan and Leah walked over to William and Ryan and knelt down. We circled the family as Jordan asked them, "How would you like to live next door to Aunt Meredith and Uncle Brad?" That meant living next door to their cousins! They had found their home.

I have been told that cancer can divide families. I believe that because the pain is so deep, and the battle so hard and long, it wounds everyone. But I know that God can take deep sorrows and draw people together even more closely than they might have been. Inviting God into the middle of the mess made all the difference.

We celebrated! Wayne's birthday, clean scans, and a new home! To top off the week, Stephanie wanted to go on the two hour zip line tour. Meredith agreed to join her, and then Justin said he was up for that and would give up a round of golf to go with them. Somehow, they talked me into it. There were ten lines scattered on the mountain. It was a picture-perfect day and the walk through the woods to each platform was stunning. That was the easy part. Stepping off that first platform into space conflicted with every sensible bone in my body! But I couldn't let my kids down, and by the last long ride, I swung upside down and spread my arms out in joy!

*****

Those weeks of rest and laughter rebuilt both body and spirit. Spirit faster than body! Wayne was still very thin when we again journeyed to St. Mary's on August 12. Again I waited for the doctor's report and tried to corral my anxious thoughts. Like recalcitrant toddlers my thoughts jumped and scattered drawn to the bristles of anxiety.

Finally, the doctor in his familiar green surgical scrubs swept into the conference room and announced, "The stent is out. Everything looks good. The kidney is functioning." In just a few words a heavy burden was lifted.

The final piece of good news that summer came a week later when Wayne went to Lemmen-Holton for blood work, and his oncologist said, "You are doing well. Enjoy yourself. We'll do another scan the end of September."

Pondering

How can food, family, simple vacation time be key to rebuilding the body and the spirit?.

Chapter 25

Autumn Anguish

My sheep listen to my voice; I know them, and they follow me. I give them eternal life, and they shall never perish; no one can snatch them out of my hand. John 10:27-28

"There is a shadow on or in your pancreas. The Merkel could be back, or it could be pancreatic cancer, or it could be a shadow."

September 23 the sun shone and we had planned to walk the streets of Grand Rapids, enjoying Art Prize (an amazing international art competition and festival drawing thousands of people to our city). But first we had to stop by Lemmen-Holton for the results of Wayne's latest, routine scan.

Since August 12 when the stent had been removed, Wayne had been growing stronger. Summer weather had lingered through September, and we relished the warmth and sense of renewed health. We had reveled in days without treatments and pushed away thoughts of cancer. I had joined a Bible study again and began tentatively writing our story, not realizing, or maybe not wanting to think, that there were more chapters to unfold. Our defenses were down. Neither of us had braced ourselves for this possibility.

We didn't go to Art Prize, we didn't walk the sunny streets, we went home to grieve and regroup. We had learned what such a finding would mean: more tests, decisions, treatments, a battering to Wayne's body that was just starting to recover, and more stress on our children and grandchildren.

The car was silent. Wayne usually has music playing. His taste is eclectic: gospel, rock, country, praise songs. That day, he turned the music off. I knew I had to text the kids. I knew I needed to breathe. That's all I could do at first, just breathe. I wanted to be encouraging, but I could not think of anything. Finally a verse flitted through my thoughts: *Give thanks in all circumstances, for this is God's will for you in Christ Jesus* (I Thessalonians 5:18).

I reached over to touch Wayne's shoulder, "It's only one spot. They caught it early. I'm thankful for that. We'll figure this out."

I texted and pushed down the volcanic rage I felt. Apparently, not very successfully.

3:16 the next morning I woke up, my eyelids still swollen from crying myself to sleep. *"For God so loved . . ."* oh yeah—*this is how you love us!?!*

Sitting alone in the family room, I wept . . . and raged. I could not read. My prayers were fractured. I wrestled with God. Finally, my eyes fell on Max Lucado's devotional book. It fell open to "God's Call to Courage." *We aren't to be oblivious to the overwhelming challenges that life brings. We're to counterbalance them with long looks at God's accomplishments.*[5]

God held me close like a flailing child until I could hear His whispers, *Yes, I love you and Wayne dearly. I am still in control. I will give you peace and courage and hope. I am faithful. I won't let you go.*

The next few weeks filled with doctor appointments and plans to return to Mayo Clinic. Skirmishes with anger, frustration, and sadness continued, though not as severe as that hour of rage. On September 30, I wrote in my journal: *I'm so sick of cancer robbing his health, our finances, our time and involvement with family, and ministry, and work . . . . Sometimes I want to explode. God please take the resentment and anger. Help us know your will. Fill me. I'm empty.*

Again the scriptures gave direction. I read James, one of my dad's favorite Bible passages. It's all about trials designed to make us more like Jesus, and how I should respond to them. *Thank you, Heavenly Father, for hearing me and helping me. Strengthen us to endure and honor you.*

Splashes of red, orange, rust, and crimson filled the trees and soothed our spirits as we drove the many miles to Rochester. Thursday, Wayne had another scan which revealed the spot was in his pancreas. Monday, he was in pre-op for an endoscopic ultrasound and biopsy. His nurse Paul performed his tasks with kindness, then paused before he left, "I'm praying for you." Prayers lifted by so many. Gifts of grace showered down on us.

The results revealed a return of the Merkel cancer. Radiation was recommended, and it could be done in Grand Rapids.

We met with more doctors. Some say so little. Perhaps they don't realize silence can be discouraging. For me words are the sunshine and water for hope. Our hope can shrivel in the drought of uncertainty and the dark nights of waiting. Words have power to encourage and comfort a wounded spirit. People think I am strong, but most of the time I feel fractured.

*****

Chicago was calling my name. Hannah had an October birthday. It was her turn to celebrate her seventh birthday with her mama and grandma at the American Girl store in Chicago and stay overnight at the Embassy Suites. The tradition had started five years earlier with our oldest granddaughter, Grace. She had told me how much she loved American Girl dolls and hoped to have one someday. She was six at the time.

I looked them up, flinched at the price, and turned to my high school students. "Any of you have American Girl dolls?"

Faces lit up in my Creative Writing class. Wait, these were seniors. Why all the smiles? I told them about Grace and asked what they thought about my promising her one when she was ten.

Then the stories flew. It didn't take long for them to convince me that seven was the perfect age to get one. And, a trip to Chicago with me would be a memory maker. That afternoon I called Stephanie and a family tradition began. Each year I returned with the next seven year old.

Hannah had been anticipating her trip for years. She had listened to her cousin Grace, and the next year her sister Lauren, and the next her cousin Aubrey, and finally her cousin Ashlyn. Each shared their memories and showed her the pictures of their special trip. How could I let her down, but how could I go?

Wayne had an important meeting with the radiologist, someone we didn't know and I should be there. Wayne did not agree. I argued that Hannah would understand, but I hated to disappoint my sweet, quiet granddaughter who on her sixth birthday had just wanted to spend the day with me, no gift! (What a day we had at Meijer Gardens that year!)

*****

Every Monday night for over thirty years, Wayne has met up with Dan. It started when they were both managers at Russ' Restaurant and continued after they retired. Dan was a prayer warrior for Wayne and often texted him verses and words of encouragement.

"Elaine doesn't want to go to Chicago because I have another appointment," Wayne shared the Monday night just a day before I had to cancel or decide to go.

"I'll go with you." Dan didn't just offer, Wayne told me, he insisted.

When he came home and told me, a wave of relief gave me the permission I needed.

Dan called my cell as Meredith, Hannah, and I rode the train to Chicago. He gave me the details I craved. The "young" doctor (I had looked him up.) had trained at Mayo Clinic under Wayne's radiologist there. He knew Dr. B., Wayne's Mayo oncologist, and he was happy to consult with them. Dan even shared that Wayne had quipped to the doctor, "After your reunion, I hope you remember to discuss my case."

The next twenty-four hours were an emotional transfusion. The sky was blue, the temperature ideal for walking, and three generations bonded in a special way. After Hannah picked her perfect match and named her Rebecca, I suggested we could call this Rebecca's birthday. Hannah disagreed, "No, it's her adoption day!" (Just like her brother's.)

*****

Our prayer list of fellow cancer fighters grew through the fall. One way both Wayne and I had changed was in the intensity of our prayers for fellow travelers. We knew what a difference prayers were making on our journey. We longed to share the comfort and encouragement we had received.

We treasured our prayer partners and the kindnesses that seemed to arrive at just the right time: the gift card for a restaurant in Rochester, a gift of $100 during our five-week stay there, and a beautiful handmade afghan and prayer shawl on our return. Flowers, cards with encouragement, text messages, a cup of coffee with a friend brightened the path on our cancer journey. Each gift reminded us God was with us through His people. We felt grateful, humbled, and challenged to reach out more.

Pondering

Have you wrestled with God? How did He speak to you? Has your journey increased your awareness of the needs of fellow travelers?

[5]Lucado, Max. Live Loved: Experiencing God's Presence in Everyday Life. (Nashville: Thomas Nelson, 2011), 134.

Chapter 26

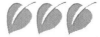

Golf, Gifts, God with Us, Emmanuel

These commandments that I give you today are to be on your hearts. Impress them on your children. Talk about them when you sit at home and when you walk along the rode . . . . Numbers 6:6-7

"I'm going golfing with Warren and Nels!" Wayne announced after his final radiation treatment on December 10! December 10 in Michigan rarely finds anyone on the golf course. That gift came wrapped in sunshine.

He had tolerated the twenty-five radiation treatments well from October to December. We had even celebrated on November 22 with a halfway-there cake that Meredith had made, half covered with vanilla icing, half with chocolate.

The doctor's office told Wayne, "Your next scan is December 28. We'll probably get the results after the New Year." We knew waiting for results required patience. We had learned that much. But we had also learned a lot about choosing how to live each day we were given.

Light the advent candles of hope, love, joy, and peace. Celebrate Jesus Christ, Emmanuel, God with us.

Like many families, we have Christmas traditions that are woven into our celebration. Usually we snap a family picture *after* we each share a Bible verse that helped us during the previous year. This year Jordan and Meredith insisted we do the picture first. I've learned to be flexible so after getting no answer when I asked "Why?" I just found my spot and smiled.

The youngest grandchild begins, reciting a verse, usually with a Bible on his or her lap even if they can't read. The tradition encourages each person to simply share a verse, and perhaps add why or when they chose that verse. These are my favorite moments, holy moments, sometimes, shiny-eyed tearful moments.

Justin was next, but for the first time, did not have a verse to share. *Okay, let it go,* I told myself. Jordan, Leah, Meredith, Brad, Stephanie, Paul each smiled and shook their heads as if they did not have a verse. Now I was getting confused. Wayne shrugged and shared his.

"You'll need this." Then everyone laughed and Stephanie handed me a tissue box,

"We decided to share our verses this way this year." Jordan was plugging wires from his laptop into the television.

The lights were dimmed . . . .

It was December 26, 2015, the night our family gathered to celebrate Christmas together. It was December 26, 1969, when we had promised each other, ". . . to love and cherish, for better or for worse, for richer or poorer, in sickness and in health as long as we both shall live."

Music began and I reached for Wayne's hand. *What is the Measure of a Life?* appeared in white letters on a black background. Wayne's fingers tightened around mine. Through music, words, and pictures our children shared their verses, their love, and precious memories. I wasn't the only one who reached for a tissue that night.

Two days, later Wayne was back at Lemmen-Holton for another scan.

Pondering

Here are the verses our children shared that very special night. Perhaps one of them will encourage you today: Galatians 5:22-23, Joshua 24:15, Luke 10:27, Ecclesiastes 4:9-12, Romans 8:28, Philippians 4:6-7, and I Corinthians 13.

Chapter 27

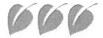

The News and Knee-Time

"I have revealed and saved and proclaimed—you are my witnesses,"
declares the Lord, "that I am God." Isaiah 43:12

No news on January 1, or 2, or 3, or 4 . . . Preparing for whatever God decided, we took time to reflect on the past year, the unexpected year. We had learned that with unexpected pain and fear the best response is to trust God more. Trust that He is at work; trust that He will provide unexpected blessings like the intensity of our children and grandchildren's love and support.

Recognize His hand: on the family doctor who did not take a "wait and see" approach, but searched for answers quickly; and His hand in the trip to Mayo, the perfect timing with every detail covered, the plane, the pilot. Acknowledge the strength He gave us to face giants.

Be grateful for the grace of our Pastor Jim and the God-messages he brought us from Hebrews and Joshua. Give thanks for all the caring medical people from Metro to St. Mary's to Lemmen-Holton, to Mayo.

Be amazed with the faithful prayers of so many including family, friends, acquaintances, and even strangers. Express gratitude for the neighbors who cut the grass, trimmed the edges, raked the beach. Give praises for the songs, the Psalms, the devotionals, the moments of joy. The list went on and on and every one of them reminded us, God so loved us that our hearts overflowed.

It was the beginning of January, the morning of a sunny winter day in Michigan. I had logged on to Wayne's patient portal as I had learned to do and had for the past five mornings, but this time, the report was there.

Wayne was sitting on the sofa having devotions. My heart began to race, my breathing became shallow. I forced myself to take a deep breath and before I read, prayed, *Father, have mercy. Your will be done.*

I plowed through medical terms and at the bottom saw the news. I gasped.

"What?" Wayne asked. Then he saw my face and came over.

"Read this! Does this say what I think it says?"

Wayne's eyes scanned the paragraph I pointed to, and tears filled his eyes. "I was braced for bad news. This, this is . . . so good." He lifted his hand to Heaven.

Something nagged at me. "But are we reading it correctly? I'm going to call the nurse."

Wayne agreed that neither of us understood every word, and there could be something we were missing. I had to leave a message on the recording that promised to return my call as soon as possible.

An hour later my precious niece Nicole stopped by. She was visiting from California and had been one of her Uncle Wayne's staunch prayer warriors. My phone rang as they hugged.

"To answer the question you left: Yes, this is a very good report. The doctor will explain everything when you come in in two days."

"Thank you, I wasn't sure." My voice cracked with emotion.

"I understand. I'm happy for you."

"Hey, Nicole. You can be the first to know. I haven't texted the family yet. Wanted to be sure. Uncle Wayne just got a good report on his scan! Praise God!"

We huddled for a moment in a tight embrace. "I have to tell the family!" I stepped into our bedroom so Wayne and Nicole could talk, and I could share our joy with family and friends. Ten minutes later I came back.

"Nicole, would you run some errands with me?" Something prompted me to ask. I had learned more and more to trust the promptings of the Spirit, not to argue.

"Let's go. I have time. We can visit more when I get back. You'll be here, right?"

"Sure," Wayne assured her. Then he whispered in my ear, "Thanks, I need some knee-time."

Pondering

Have you ever taken time to reflect on God's goodness in seasons of struggle? Ever need some time alone just to get on your knees?

10 Months Later

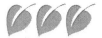

Epilogue   Wayne: I Just Bought my Last Broom

*The Lord watches over you—the Lord is your shade at your right hand . .
. . Psalm 121:5*

A few months before I was diagnosed with cancer, I was doing some
chores around the house. I went to the garage to get my broom. It was a
pathetic sight, that twenty-five year old broom. It had a wooden handle
and straw bristles that were half gone and so curled you couldn't lean it
against the wall without it falling over. I thought, *Wayne, you cheap
Dutchman, go buy yourself a new broom!* Before I could talk myself out
of it, I jumped in my car and was off to Home Depot.

They had nice brooms there. I chose a blue one with a plastic handle
and plastic bristles that were cut at a diagonal. On my way home it
dawned on me that I had probably just bought my last broom. After all, if
this one lasts twenty-five years, I'll be ninety years old!

A few days later I was patching some cracks in my asphalt driveway
with tar and didn't want anyone to ride over the wet repairs. With that in
mind, I laid some tools alongside the cracks, one of them being my new
broom. I'll bet you know where this is going. Sure enough, the
newspaper delivery service drove over it during the night and cracked it.

I've heard it said that God smiles when He hears about our man-made
plans. Who was I to think my broom would last twenty-five years, or
even more importantly, that I was going to live to be ninety years old?

In the Bible, God's people sang Psalm 121 for protection on their
journey to Jerusalem. I claimed that Psalm for my cancer journey.

I lift up my eyes to the mountains—
where does my help come from?
My help comes from the Lord,
the Maker of heaven and earth.

He will not let your foot slip—
He who watches over you will not slumber;
indeed, He who watches over Israel
will neither slumber nor sleep.

The Lord watches over you—
the Lord is your shade at your right hand;
the sun will not harm you by day,
nor the moon by night.

The Lord will keep you from all harm—
He will watch over your life;
the Lord will watch over your coming and going
both now and forevermore.

I was on a journey before the cancer, but it didn't seem quite as clear then. We are all on a journey and mine is not that much different from yours. Cancer is not fun. There are times when I am weak, times when I am strong, times when I am anxious, times when I am at peace. I know this journey would be a lot harder without my wife, my children, and my grandchildren, who give me great joy, my friends and prayer partners who continually lift me up in prayer, and especially my God, *who neither slumbers nor sleeps.*

I don't know where you are in your journey, but as I write these words, I have just had my third clear scan. I don't know what the future holds, but I know who holds it, and I am so grateful for the healing so far. And, oh yeah, my new replacement broom is now two and a half years old.

Lessons and strategies that we learned to help Three Generations Fight Cancer Together

We learned to:

Take time to grieve,

Pray,

Share the news. We found ways to communicate by phone, email, text, Facebook,

Touch, hold hands, hold each other, and hug often,

Ask for prayer,

Accept and consider advice, listen well,

Ask questions,

Take time to do fun things,

Say "I love you" often,

Express appreciation,

Keep records,

Check our insurance policy especially before we went out of network,

Go to appointments,

Let the children and grandchildren be part of the solution,

Respect each person's way of processing the news and responding,

Choose a Psalm, a song, and a symbol as a reminder of God's faithfulness,

Research what else might help, educate ourselves,

Read the Bible and devotionals,

Get a second opinion,

Worship together,

Celebrate little things and big things,

Let people into the story,

Let Wayne (the patient) make decisions, express needs,

Be flexible,

Reach out to a wider circle of support,

Set priorities: What matters?

Remember it is a marathon, not a sprint,

Savor something good every day,

Reach out to others and help them,

Take time to recover,

Go to the elders for prayer,

Accept the kindness of friends, neighbors, and even strangers,

Make a halfway-there cake,

Get on our knees,

Celebrate good news,

Remain vigilant,

Praise and thank God,

Trust Him in all things.

*****

Our game plan for keeping track of information:
- The green notebook that fit in my purse, used at every appointment. I recorded the date, the doctor, the comments, and the results that were given.
- A 3-ring binder for insurance papers. I punched holes in the insurance papers and saved them in chronological order.
- A second 3-ring binder for medical information which held:
    - A page for each month of the year where I recorded every test and appointment. This proved to be especially helpful when doctors asked questions like, "When was your last scan?" "When was your last chemo treatment?" You would think that would all be on their computer screen, but my records were often a quicker reference.
    - Dividers which I labeled and used for the medical papers we received. (Use the hole-puncher.)
    - Two plastic business card holder sheets with 3 hole punches to keep all the names and phone numbers of the

doctors, treatment centers, and contact people. This proved to be a valuable resource for quick reference when I needed a phone number.

Gratitude and Blessings

May the Lord repay you for what you have done. May you be richly rewarded by the Lord. Ruth 2:12

There are some debts that I cannot repay; they are too big for me. Thankfully, I can ask God to pay them for me by blessing the people who have offered priceless gifts to us both on our cancer journey and our writing journey. So dear extended family, friends, acquaintances, and even strangers, I thank you and bless you in Jesus' name.

To all who prayed, sent cards, text messages, Facebook greetings, I cannot begin to list all of you, but God knows you by name, and I ask Him to bless you richly. Nor can I name all who showed us a kindness, but God knows you and may He bless your socks off!

To all the doctors who helped Wayne—We offer our deepest gratitude for all you did and do for him as well as so many other cancer patients. To all the medical people, from doctors to nurses, to technicians, to staff who work with diligence and compassion in the fight against cancer, may God continue to bless and strengthen you. Thank you Metro Hospital, St. Mary's Hospital, Lemmen-Holton Cancer Pavilion, Spectrum Hospital, and Mayo Clinic.

To Calvary Church: our pastor Jim Samra, the visiting team, our small group, Women's Bible Study, Arlene Timmer, the elders, and fellow members, the prayer warriors—Thank you for all you do for the Kingdom; all you did for us.

Thank you to all who blessed this manuscript with your insights and encouragement. Writing and publishing a book brought me on a wonderful journey of learning. The following people were my teachers, guides, and encouragers. My deepest gratitude:

To Barb Opperwall, Lorilee Reimer Cracker, and Cindy Bultema, who read the first few chapters and said, "Keep writing."

To Word Weavers of Holland/Zeeland led by Denise Vredevoogd, strangers who became dear friends giving me courage, honest feedback, and concrete suggestions. And deep gratitude to Sharon Ruff for permission to share her beautiful poem, *For You I Write.*

To my readers who contributed encouragement, editing suggestions, proofreading, and insights: Carla and Tom Mockabee, Kathy Richert, Susan Brems, Kristen Ward, Fayth Steensma, Dan Post, Barb Opperwall, and Lorilee Reimer Cracker. Thank you for your diligent help. Any mistakes are mine.

To my fellow book lovers in our Laughing Ladies Literary Club, for your love and laughter and prayers: Marybeth Bush, Karen Miedema, Helen Bell, Suzanne Greydanus, Jami Dunbar, Bethany DenBoer, JulieAnn Teunis, Fayth Steensma, Barb Opperwall, Kim Groenenboom, Jobi Hasse.

To the Christian writing conferences that taught me so much: Calvin College's Festival of Faith and Writing, Carol Kent's Speak Up Conference, Maranatha Writers' Conference, and the Breathe Christian Writers' Conference.

To Cheri Cowell, Bob Ousnamer, Kristen Veldhuis and the team at EA Books Publishing who guided me through the publication process.

To each one of you who helped me on this writing adventure: Thank you for your blessings to me.

Overflowing love and thanks to our children: Stephanie and Paul, Meredith and Brad, Jordan and Leah, and Justin; and to our grandchildren: Grace, Lauren, Aubrey, Ashlyn, William, Hannah, Ryan, and Andrew. You traveled with us. You gave us your love and support. And then you added your writing, memories, and blessings to share our story. Jesus shines through you. And a special shout-out to our son Justin, who answered every call for computer, printer, and technology help with patience and expertise. You might have saved your mom's sanity.

And to Wayne, my love, who weeps with me, laughs with me, and daily teaches me to savor life. I love you.

Above all, to God from whom every good gift comes, I am eternally grateful. He is faithful through every challenge.

RESOURCES

We did not use every idea we read. What we did do is pray, study, and implement what we felt led to try. We learned a lot and were blessed. Perhaps some of these will help you.

Bollinger, Ty M. *The Truth about Cancer: What You Need to Know about Cancer's History, Treatment, and Prevention.* Carlsbad, CA: Hay House, Inc., 2016.

Dobson, Ed. *Prayers and Promises When Facing a Life-Threatening Illness.* Grand Rapids, MI: Zondervan, 2007.

Feinberg, Margaret. *Fight Back With Joy.* Brentwood, TN: Worthy Books, 2015.

Gibbs, Terri. *Joy for the Journey.* Dallas: Word Publishing, Inc., 1997.

Katz, MD, MPH, David L., and Stacey Colino. *Disease Proof: Slash Your Risk of Heart Disease, Cancer, Diabetes, and More.* New York: Penguin Group, 2013.

Kelfer, Russell. *Wait: A Journey to Discovering the Heart of God.* Fort Worth, TX: Brownlow Corporation, 2003.

Lucado, Max. *Live Loved: Experiencing God's Presence in Everyday Life.* Nashville: Thomas Nelson, 2011.

Meyer, Joyce. *Battlefied of the Mind.* 2nd ed. New York: FaithWords, 2011.

Niequist, Shauna. *Savor.* Grand Rapids, MI: Zondervan, 2015.

Servan-Schreiber, MD, PhD, David. *Anticancer: A New Way of Life.* 2nd ed. New York: Viking Penguin, 2009.

Sorensen, Susan, and Laura Geist. *Praying Through Cancer: Set Your Heart Free from Fear.* Nashville, Thomas Nelson, 2006.

Ten Elshof, Phyllis. *What Cancer Cannot Do.* Grand Rapids, MI: Zondervan, 2006.

Turner, Ph.D., Kelly A. *Radical Remission: Surviving Cancer Against All Odds*. New York: HarperCollins, 2014.

Voskamp, Ann. *One Thousand Gifts*. Grand Rapids, MI: Zondervan, 2010.

Young, Sarah. *Jesus Calling*. Nashville, TN: Thomas Nelson, 2004.

Websites

American Cancer Society. Google. /www.cancer.org/research/cancer-facts-.

Axe, Josh. Axe Wellness, LLC. Google.

Calvary Church. www.calvarygr.org.

Heidelberg Catechism/Christian Reformed Church. Google https://www.crcna.org/.

Mayo Foundation for Medical Education and Research (MFMER). www.mayoclinic.org/.

Mercola, Joseph. Google. www.mercola.com/.
Nikken. http://www.nikken.com/.

Made in the USA
Lexington, KY
19 July 2017